GENETIC ENGINEERING, CHRISTIAN VALUES AND CATHOLIC TEACHING

GENETIC ENGINEERING, CHRISTIAN VALUES AND CATHOLIC TEACHING

Paul Flaman

PAULIST PRESS
New York/Mahwah, N.J.

Book design by Joseph E. Petta

Cover design by Valerie Petro

Library of Congress Cataloging-in-Publication Data

Flaman, Paul
Genetic engineering : Christian values and Catholic teaching / Paul Flaman.
    p.   cm.
  Includes bibliographical references and index.
  ISBN 0-8091-4089-6
    1. Genetic engineering—Moral and ethical aspects. 2. Genetic engineering—Religious aspects—Christianity. 3. Genetic engineering—Religious aspects—Catholic Church. I. Title.
QH442 .F525 2002
174'.25—dc21

                                                              2002012512

Published by Paulist Press
997 Macarthur Boulevard
Mahwah, New Jersey 07430

www.paulistpress.com

Printed and bound
in Canada

Contents

Abbreviations:

AIDS	Acquired Immunodeficiency Syndrome
AMA	American Medical Association
CBC	Canadian Broadcasting Corporation
CCC	*Catechism of the Catholic Church*
CDF	Congregation for the Doctrine of the Faith
CHAC	Catholic Health Association of Canada
CHAUSA	Catholic Health Association of the United States of America
CIA	United States Central Intelligence Agency
CMA	Canadian Medical Association
DNA	Deoxyribonucleic Acid
DOE	Department of Energy
EB	*The New Encyclopedia Britannica: Macropaedia* (1975)
ELSI	The National Human Genome Research Institute's Ethical, Legal, and Social Implications Program
FBI	United States Federal Bureau of Investigation
FDA	The United States Food and Drug Administration
GMO	Genetically Modified Organism
HGP	Human Genome Project
HIV	Human Immunodeficiency Virus
IVF	In Vitro Fertilization
LRCC	Law Reform Commission of Canada
MRCC	Medical Research Council of Canada
NBAC	National Bioethics Advisory Commission
NFB	National Film Board of Canada
NFP	Natural Family Planning
NIH	United States National Institutes of Health
NSGC	National Society of Genetic Counselors, Inc.
PGD	Preimplantation Genetic Diagnosis
PKU	Phenylketonuria
PTO	United States Patents and Trademark Office
RAFI	Rural Advancement Foundation International

RCNRT	Canada's Royal Commission on New Reproductive Technologies
SRT	Society, Religion and Technology Project of the Church of Scotland
UNESCO	United Nations Educational, Scientific and Cultural Organization
U.S.	United States of America
USCC	United States Conference of Catholic Bishops
WMA	World Medical Association

To Jesus Christ, fully human and fully divine,
who shares our human genome and is the light of the world.

Abstract:

Genetic Engineering, Christian Values and Catholic Teaching by Paul
Flaman aims to provide a good overview of the ethical issues faced
by many individuals and our society as a whole today in the whole
area of genetics. This book is intended to provide a resource for
teachers: science and religion teachers from grades seven to twelve,
and university instructors in bioethics and other related fields. The
book is also intended to be used as reading material for university or
college level students including nursing students and seminarians.
Because of the issues treated, the book may be of interest to a wider
audience as well. The book's Introduction provides a brief overview
of major developments from Gregor Mendel to the Eugenics Movement to the Human Genome Project, genetic therapy and cloning.
Chapter 1 discusses ethical issues related to the genetic engineering
of plants and animals. Topics treated include agribusiness, ecological
concerns, biological warfare, genetically modified food, transgenic
animals, cloning and patenting life forms. Chapter 2 discusses ethical
issues related to the genetic engineering of human beings. Topics
treated include genetic testing, counseling, therapy, enhancement,
cloning and eugenics. In Chapters 1 and 2 the main ethical posi-
tions, including that of Catholic teaching, are presented. Chapter 3
discusses some major views on plant, animal and human life today.
The author's view is included in the light of the Christian themes of
creation, sin, redemption and the incarnation of Jesus Christ. Chapter 4 provides some additional ethical analysis and reflection, noting
areas of widespread agreement and major controversies today related
to genetics and values. These are reflected upon comparing a few
different ethical approaches, including consequentialist, feminist and
official Catholic. While taking an ecumenical approach, the author

supports Catholic teaching, arguing for a consistent life and relational ethics in the light of Christian values.

Acknowledgments:

First of all, I would like to thank Mervyn Lynch, a leader for years with the Edmonton Catholic schools, who felt a need for this kind of book as a resource for teachers and others. He invited me to write this book and has been very supportive. I would also like to thank a few people at the University of Alberta: Dr. Rachel Wevrick, a medical geneticist, Elmar Prenner, a biochemist, and Catholic bioethicists Dr. Rebecca Davis Mathias (St. Joseph's College) and Dr. Eric Kilbreath (formerly with St. Joseph's College Ethics Centre), who offered some valuable suggestions for improving the book. I would like to thank as well Fr. Eric Reichers and Sr. Mary Lou Cranston, leading Catholic educators, and my wife Maggie, for their support. Finally, I would like to thank Fr. Joseph Scott, C.S.P., and others of Paulist Press for their contributions to preparing this book for publication.

Notes and sources are named briefly within the text. More complete information on these sources is found in the References *section at the conclusion of the book.*

Introduction:
An Overview of Some
Major Developments

Even from ancient times certain facts about heredity have been known. It was observed that children resemble their parents and grandparents, and that certain typical traits are transmitted from generation to generation. For thousands of years humans have been selectively breeding plants and animals to eliminate or enhance certain traits. The ancient philosophical work, Plato's *Republic,* idealizes a society in which rulers supervise marriage and reproduction for the improvement of the human race.

In 1863 the Austrian Catholic monk Gregor Mendel, who experimented with peas, demonstrated that traits were distributed in inherited units, which were later called genes. Francis Galton, a cousin of Charles Darwin, is considered the founder of the modern movement to improve the human race by applying the laws of heredity. He coined the term *eugenics.* Between 1869 and 1889 he published several books that applied the theories of evolution, natural selection and survival of the fittest, as they were understood then, to the human race. In 1904 Galton officially launched the Eugenics Movement. He and his followers thought charitable institutions and governments protected the "unfit," of which many survived to propagate their own kind, leading to a "decay" in the human race. They thought governments should intervene to prevent the propagation of the "unfit" by forbidding their marriage, separating them from society or by forcibly sterilizing them; and to encourage and help the "superior" to propagate their kind to improve the human race (cf. Varga 1984, 75–77; and EB 1975, 6:1023).

Eugenics was seen by many leading academics, politicians and much of the public as salvation regarding many diseases, imbecility, crime, poverty and other social ills that social reform had failed to solve. Beginning in 1907 a number of states in the United States enacted sterilization laws. In 1925 the U.S. Supreme Court ruled that sterilization fell within the police powers of the state. By 1931 thirty states had passed sterilization laws and tens of thousands of American citizens had been surgically "fixed" (Rifkin 1998, 122–23). In Canada, Alberta and British Columbia enacted eugenic sterilization laws in 1928 and 1933, respectively. Before these laws were repealed in 1972 and 1973, respectively, their eugenics boards approved several thousand cases of sterilization of people deemed likely to transmit mental disorders to their offspring (LRCC 1979, 24–29).

The Eugenics Movement reached its peak in 1924 in the United States and collapsed with the stock market crash in 1929—many of the elite were now unemployed in poverty alongside others. In 1933 Hitler came to power and enacted the Hereditary Health Law, a eugenics sterilization statute that began a massive eugenics campaign. Among other atrocities, the Nazis used eugenic ideas to justify sterilizing several hundred thousand people and killing millions of people over the next twelve years. This was another major factor in the decline of the American eugenics movement (Rifkin 1998, 124–27; cf. O'Callaghan 1994, 17; and Arthur Dyck in Kilner et al. 1997, 27–28).

In the context of the Eugenics Movement one can better appreciate Aldous Huxley's *Brave New World*. This 1932 novel presents the nightmare of a future society based on an extreme application of eugenics, genetic engineering and social control (cf. Robert Wright in *Time* 1999, 51).

By the early 1950s the work of a number of scientists demonstrated that genes are made up of long molecules of deoxyribonucleic acid (DNA) composed of units of adenine (A), thymine (T), cytosine (C) and guanine (G), which are now known as nucleotides. In 1953 James Watson and Francis Crick proposed their now famous model whereby DNA is made up of two chains of nucleotides, intertwined in the form of a double helix (Roy et al. 1994, 441–42).

In the mid-1950s Dr. Bevis pioneered prenatal diagnosis using amniocentesis to predict the severity of anemia resulting from Rh incompatibility between the fetus and its mother. Several years later Dr. Liley reported the first successful intrauterine transfusion of blood to the fetus in danger of dying from Rh-incompatibility anemia. Prenatal diagnosis was first developed with truly therapeutic intentions. Some years later, however, when abortion laws became less restrictive in many countries and many came to tolerate abortion, prenatal diagnosis became more and more associated with selective abortion (Roy et al. 1994, 167–68).

By the mid-1960s the combined work of many scientists had led to deciphering the genetic code or the basic chemical logic of life.

> That logic can be summarized in four interlinked steps, somewhat as follows: The properties of living organisms result from the proteins they contain, and the human organism contains an estimated 30,000 proteins; the proteins are determined by the sequence of the amino acids of which they are constituted; the amino acid sequence, in turn, is governed by the order of the nucleotides in messenger RNA; and that order is determined by the sequence of nucleotides in the DNA of the genes. (Roy et al. 1994, 442)

With regard to this, a disorder in the sequence of nucleotides in the DNA of genes can result in a protein disorder that can cause the physical symptoms of a genetic disease. Hereditary diseases may also be due to chromosomal defects (e.g., Down's syndrome is caused by an extra 21st chromosome). With regard to hereditary diseases due to gene defects, there are several types. Some hereditary disorders are related to a single-gene defect (e.g., Tay-Sachs disease and beta-thalassemia), the expression of which may be modulated by the presence of other genes or environmental factors. Others are polygenic or related to more than one gene. In some disorders that are multifactorial, that is, they are influenced by multiple genes and environmental factors, genetic factors may only indicate a predisposition (e.g., an inherited predisposition to breast cancer) and may not mean that the person will definitely suffer from the disease. Some defective genes are recessive—a person carrying one of the genes does not have the disease (e.g., cystic fibrosis), whereas a person who has two copies of the defective gene, one from the father and one from the mother, has the disease. A genetic disease is dominant when a defective gene from either the father or mother results in the disease (e.g., Huntington's disease). Some genetic diseases are related to one of the two sex chromosomes: e.g., Duchenne muscular dystrophy is linked to the X chromosome and boys are affected if their single X chromosome carries the gene defect (Roy et al. 1994 170; Sutton 1995, 77–78; MRCC et al. 1998, 8.1).

One feature of genes is "their ability to be replicated identically and transmitted from generation to generation." But genes are also susceptible to change through a process called mutation. "Mutations may occur during the process of cell division to produce eggs and sperm, through exposure to specific environmental factors..., or as a consequence of spontaneous change." Although mutations can result in advantages to an individual and species, for example, improved speed or strength, "in many cases a change in the DNA sequence of a gene will result in malfunction of the gene and disease in the organism" (Science Council of Canada 1991, 6; cf. O'Callaghan 1994, 19).

In June 1973 the Gordon Research Conference on Nucleic Acids announced a technical innovation: recombining genes from different forms of life, which came to be known as recombinant DNA technology. This involves splicing a gene or a DNA fragment from one form of life to another, for example, from a rabbit to bacteria, and producing multiple copies by molecular cloning. Methods of gene transfer (viruses are commonly used as vectors or carriers) enable scientists to splice specific genes or DNA fragments into cells cultured in a laboratory or into the body or germ-line (ova or sperm) cells of living animals. In one experiment scientists transferred human growth hormone genes into fertilized mouse eggs, which resulted in mice double their normal size. Transgenic mice are now routinely created for research in molecular biology and genetics (Roy et al. 1994, 443; cf. MRCC et al. 1998, 8.5).

In 1980 the U.S. Supreme Court granted a patent on the first genetically engineered life form. In 1987 the Patents and Trademarks Office ruled that all genetically engineered multicellular living organisms, including animals, are potentially patentable. This includes the possibility of patenting even parts of humans but does not include patenting a whole human being. In May 1995 a large coalition of U.S. religious leaders, including more than 100 Catholic bishops, announced their opposition "to the granting of patents on animal and human genes, organs, tissues, and organisms" (Rifkin 1998, 42–65).

On October 1, 1990, the Human Genome Project (HGP) began a projected fifteen-year international undertaking involving many scientists around the world. It was estimated that it would cost some three billion U.S. dollars. The first phase of the project aimed at mapping the location of each of the tens of thousands of human genes on the forty-six human chromosomes that are paired, twenty-two autosomes, and the X and Y sex chromosomes. Initially it was estimated that there are about 100,000 human genes. In February 2001, however, two teams of scientists with the HGP and Celera Genomics respectively published studies estimating the total number of human genes to be only between 30,000 to 40,000. Some other groups, nevertheless, still think the number is higher. For example, a group at Ohio State University says that gene prediction programs tend to miss many genes. It has analyzed the same information that the HGP did and believes there may be about 80,000 genes (BioNews, May 14, 2001).

Another goal of the HGP was to sequence the complete human genome. The sequence of a gene is the complete DNA text of the gene made up of the nucleotides A, T, C and G, set out in their proper order. The DNA of the human genome has an estimated three billion of these nucleotides. The complete text of the total sequence of the human genome would fill about a thousand thousand-page telephone books. Sequencing genes, however, does not necessarily mean that we will understand the significance of the order or the functioning of the genes. A related project has also been undertaken to map, sequence and determine the function of the genes in the genomes of four so-called model organisms: the bacterium E. coli, the nematode worm, the fruit fly, and eventually the mouse. This is being done to assist interpretation of the sequence of the human genome, since "many of the genes of these smaller organisms function in ways very similar to corresponding human genes." It is expected that the HGP will facilitate research and development in a diversity of scientific fields, related commercial fields, and medicine, including diagnostic tests and genetic therapy (Roy et al. 1994, 444–45 and 447–49; cf. Colleton 1993, 1).

It was originally hoped that the HGP would sequence all human DNA by 2005. New ways to speed up the decoding process, however, have been discovered. On June 26, 2000, representatives of the HGP and the biotechnology company Celera announced the completion of the first rough draft of the entire human genome sequence. It is now expected that a fully finished sequence of all human DNA will be available by 2003 or sooner (Michael Lemonick and Dick Thompson in *Time* 1999, 28–35; BioNews June 26, 2000; HGP Information 2000).

The biological information being generated by the Human Genome Project is so great that it can only be managed by computers and stored electronically in thousands of databases around the world.

More than anything else, computers and software will be the tools for deciphering and utilizing the vast genetic resources of the Earth. This link between computers and biology is even having an effect on how many see life. For example, today cybernetic language is being used more regarding life such as speaking of living organisms as information systems and life as programmed activity. Among other things, some are projecting DNA chips and computers, including DNA supercomputers that would run a million times faster than today's most advanced supercomputers. One informed futurist, Jeremy Rifkin, thinks a major revolution in human history has begun. He refers to the twenty-first century as "The Biotech Century," a century that is likely to involve more and more genetic engineering (Rifkin 1998, Ch. 6).

In 1990 the Ethical, Legal, and Social Implications Program (ELSI) was established as an integral part of the Human Genome Project (HGP) by its U.S. planners. The purposes of the ELSI Program are to anticipate, examine and address the ethical, legal and social implications for individuals and society of mapping and sequencing the human genome; to stimulate public discussion of the issues; and to develop policy options that would assure that the information is used for the benefit of individuals and society. The ELSI Program is supported with U.S. federal HGP funds through the U.S. National Institutes of Health (NIH) and the U.S. Department of Energy (DOE). The National Human Genome Research Institute's ELSI web site (see ELSI in the References below) contains much relevant material, including news, information and events; policy and legislative activities; research, education and training opportunities; workshop/task force reports and recommendations. See also related web pages such as that of the U.S. National Bioethics Advisory Commission (NBAC).

In 1993 the Canadian government released *Proceed with Care: The Final Report of the Royal Commission on New Reproductive Technologies*. The Royal Commission's report includes many recommendations, including some regarding issues relevant to our topic such as cloning, the creation of animal/human hybrids, prenatal diagnosis, genetic therapy and genetic alteration (RCNRT 1993). In response to this report, the Canadian government initially drafted Bill C-47 (1996), which never became law, and more recently in May 2001 published *Proposals for Legislation Governing Assisted Human Reproduction: An Overview* (Health Canada 2001). Both of these proposals incorporate a number of the Royal Commission's recommendations. At the time of writing, however, Canada still has no relevant legislation in this area. In 1998 the Medical Research Council of Canada, the Natural Sciences and Engineering Research Council of Canada, and the Social Sciences and Humanities Research Council of Canada published a joint policy statement on *Ethical Conduct for Research Involving Humans.* Section 8 of this document includes a number of guidelines and regulations concerning "Human Genetic Research" (see MRCC et al. 1998).

Besides the United States and Canada, a number of other countries and organizations, including the United Nations have adopted some regulations relevant to genetic engineering issues. For example, in 1997 the United Nations Educational, Scientific and Cultural Organization adopted the Universal Declaration on the Human Genome and Human Rights (see UNESCO 1997). Several of these recommendations and regulations will be noted in the following discussion.

Before closing this introduction on genetic engineering, a few other significant developments in this field will be noted. In December 1992, Dr. French Anderson published news regarding the first successful human gene therapy experiment that he led. Two girls afflicted with adenosine deaminase (ADA) deficiency, who had received gene therapy for this deficiency since 1990, were now leading essentially normal lives. This meant that they did not have to live in a special sterile environment, a kind of bubble room. Since then a number of other gene therapy research protocols have been undertaken on diseases such as hemophilia B, cystic fibrosis and several cancers (Roy et al. 1994, 455).

In February 1997, Dr. Ian Wilmut, a Scottish scientist, announced the birth of the cloned sheep Dolly, the first clone of a higher adult mammal. This event provoked much interest and debate around the world. Many, for example, expressed opposition to the possibility of cloning humans. That this is a real possibility was reinforced in December 1998 when it was reported that scientists in Japan cloned several calves from a single adult cow (Weiss 1998). A number of other mammals have been cloned since (Rogers 2000). Recently there has also been much debate about cloning human embryos to provide stem cells for research which some hope will lead to new cures for diseases such as Parkinson's disease, multiple sclerosis and diabetes. On January 22, 2001, the House of Lords approved a controversial law that will allow British scientists to clone human embryos for medical research (The Associated Press London 2001). The possibility of cloning human embryos for reproductive or "therapeutic" purposes, like other possibilities of genetic engineering, raises the important ethical question of whether or not we should attempt to do whatever we have the means to do.

This introduction has provided a brief overview of a number of the major developments regarding genetics and genetic engineering. In the following we will consider some of the main ethical issues with regard to the genetic engineering of plants, animals and human beings. Among other things, the presentation will include some reflections in the light of some widely-held human values, Christian values and relevant Catholic teachings.

Chapter One

Genetic Engineering of Plants and Animals

For centuries human beings have been selectively breeding plants and animals, for example, choosing certain boars to mate certain sows to produce leaner pig meat over many generations. Few have questioned the ethics of this. Is the genetic engineering of plants and animals significantly different, and if so, why? Much is already happening with regard to the genetic engineering of plants and animals. For example, some genetically modified crops have already been produced. Inserting the gene for human growth hormone into mice embryos has resulted in mice double their normal size. These "super" mice are now reproducing themselves. Mice are being used in much genetic research seeking cures for many forms of cancer and other diseases. Genetic engineering may soon lead to the production of many foods and proteins, and more pharmacological products, in factories. Other hopes for genetic engineering include producing cows or other mammals whose milk includes valuable pharmaceutical properties, more ecological fuels, and organisms to get rid of certain wastes or pollutants. Much research is at present taking place with regard to the genetic engineering of plants and animals. We are likely to see many significant

11

developments in this area. On the one hand, this growing field promises many benefits to human beings. On the other hand, many are concerned about significant risks of harm to human beings and the environment.

1.A. Agribusiness, Ecological Concerns, Biological Warfare

Genetic science and technology are already being used for both genetic testing and engineering of plants and animals. Concerning genetic testing there is a worldwide effort to map the genomes, for example, of important crops such as wheat and corn, so that strains can be tested for their gene content compared to their pest resistance, and so forth. Another example is genetically testing grapes used for wine production to strive for consistency among wines (Wevrick 1999). Efforts are also being made to genetically engineer plants and animals to produce more protein or meat or milk, and so forth. For example, C.S. Prakash, director of the Center for Plant Biotechnology Research at Tuskegee University in Alabama, and his team of researchers have developed "a sweet potato with five times the amount of protein of a normal sweet potato." Such an improvement can benefit millions of people in Africa and elsewhere "for whom tubers are a dietary staple" (Wooden 2001). Genetically engineered plants and animals may also grow quicker or reach maturity quicker. Research is already being conducted and attempts are being made, for example, to engineer mammals whose milk contains valuable medicinal properties for sufferers from emphysema, and plants that have certain desirable qualities (e.g., tomatoes that stay firm longer, tobacco plants with inserted human genes that will produce proteins to treat juvenile diabetes and Crohn's disease, etc.) or are more resistant to frost, drought, salinity, certain diseases, herbicides, and the like (SRT 1998, "Animal and Plant Genetic Engineering"; The Canadian Press 1999; Bruce

1998, Ch. 2). The U.S. Food and Drug Administration is already supervising clinical trials of some of these products (Yoon 2000; see also FDA).

Unpredictable risks of perhaps even very serious and devastating consequences to the earth's ecosystem, to our environment and to ourselves, are among the major concerns of many people, including many scientists and ethicists, with regard to the genetic engineering of plants and animals. Some speak of "genetic pollution," that is, introducing genetically modified organisms into the environment of which some might have no natural enemies, become uncontrolled and seriously upset the ecosystem. Since living genetically engineered organisms can reproduce and migrate, they may pose far greater long-term risks to the environment than petrochemicals. Some genetically modified viruses or microorganisms, for example, that are either released into or escape into the ecosystem, could result in new diseases that could be devastating to human beings and/or other species of life.

A few examples of research already underway or being considered in this area include the following. In one experiment researchers introduced the human AIDS virus genome into mouse embryos, resulting in a number of mice in subsequent generations carrying the HIV virus. While this research was undertaken to facilitate the study of AIDS, some scientists have warned that the AIDS virus in mice could combine with other mouse viruses and perhaps result in a more virulent AIDS virus that might spread by "novel routes," including through the air. In another experiment researchers deleted the genetic instructions for making ice from a bacterium that contributes to much frost damage for farmers. If these modified "ice-minus" bacteria could replace on a large scale their natural counterparts, this could have considerable commercial benefits in preventing much frost damage. Since some scientists have shown that this same bacterium plays a key role in triggering rainfall, there is concern that if this happened on a large scale that it could have long-term effects on worldwide precipitation patterns.

Research is also underway to engineer predator insects to prey on noxious insects, fish that are more disease resistant or which can live in colder waters, and crops that are resistant to certain pests or herbicides. Although the plan may be to raise such fish with certain competitive advantages in contained fish tanks, in the past there have been accidental escapes into open waters due to unanticipated flooding. This could cause havoc in aquatic ecosystems. Transgenic crops with competitive advantages may lead to the natural development of super pests or their modified genes may pass over through cross-pollination to weedy relatives creating superweeds. Among other things, some scientists are considering the possibility of producing a genetically engineered enzyme that destroys lignin that makes wood rigid. While this could have great commercial advantages in cleaning up wastes from paper mills or in producing energy, if the enzyme migrated offsite, it could destroy millions of acres of forests (see Rifkin 1998, Ch. 3, for more details regarding these and some other examples; and Bruce 1998, Ch. 2).

A number of large corporations are hiring scientists to genetically engineer new or modified transgenic species. Some of these are being introduced into the environment with little risk assessment. In general, these corporations tend to look to short-term profits without spending much money on long-term risk assessment to the environment, ecosystem and human beings. The insurance industry will not insure the release of genetically engineered organisms into the environment because the industry lacks a risk assessment science. Global life-science companies are expected to introduce thousands of genetically engineered organisms into the environment in the coming century. Although these may be harmless in many cases, history has shown that every new technology has some harmful effects (Rifkin 1998, Ch. 3). In light of this, Dr. Donald Bruce and professors John Eldridge and Joyce Tait, for example, call for a more precautionary approach to risk assessment regarding potential new and radical biotechnologies for which we do not have sound data to establish the range of risks. They also think there should be input from a wider set of people and more public debate than has typically been the case (see SRT 1998, "Genetic Risk Regulation, Society and Ethics"; and Bruce 1998, Ch. 7).

In a document on the ecological crisis, Pope John Paul II, among other things expresses concern regarding the risks of genetic engineering, saying in part:

> We are not yet in a position to assess the biological disturbance that could result from indiscriminate genetic manipulation and from the unscrupulous development of new forms of plant and animal life....It is evident to all that in any area as delicate as this, indifference to fundamental ethical norms, or their rejection, would lead mankind to the very threshold of self-destruction.
>
> *Respect for life...is the ultimate guiding norm for any sound economic, industrial or scientific progress.*
>
> ...certain underlying principles, which, while respecting the legitimate autonomy and the specific competence of those involved, can direct research towards adequate and lasting solutions....*no peaceful society can afford to neglect either respect for life or the fact that there is an integrity to creation.* (John Paul II 1989, n. 7)

The Vatican's Pontifical Academy for Life (October 1999) has concluded that the genetic engineering of plants and animals can involve advantages and may help to solve human problems like world hunger. Bishop Elio Sgreccia of the academy says, "The risks should be carefully followed through openness, analysis and controls, but without a sense of alarm...We cannot agree with the position of some groups that say it is against the will of God to meddle with the genetic make-up of plants and animals." The environmental risks of genetic modifications should be evaluated on a case-by-case basis (Thavis 1999, 1).

In order to preserve the bounties we now enjoy, Rachel Wevrick, a geneticist, thinks we as a community need to look more at the long-term consequences not only of genetic engineering, but also at all sorts of other kinds of engineering and agricultural practices. For example, the cattle industry "has been using antibiotics routinely in cattle for many years," which has had a "negative long-term impact on the health of the cattle and the people who eat the meat and drink the milk, perhaps contributing to antibiotic resistance in people" (Wevrick 1999).

It should also be noted that the genetic engineering of plants and animals does not only involve issues concerning risks to the environment, to plants and animals themselves, and to the health and life of human beings. According to Tom Wilkie they also involve issues regarding the distribution of power among human beings and the powerlessness of some. For example, genetically engineered seeds which produce greater yields may drive smaller farmers out of business since these seeds are more expensive. Seeds engineered to resist certain herbicides, if farmers buy them, will result in the concentration of the agri-seeds and chemicals business in the hands of a few high-tech companies (Wilkie 1998, 996).

"Terminator" seeds are being genetically engineered by large multinational companies such as Monsanto. These seeds are designed to be sterile unless activated by a chemical which the company sells. These companies argue that such seeds will prevent genetic pollution and allow them a return on their investment. Many critics, however, fear that such developments could make farmers even more dependent on large multinational seed and chemical companies, and that this technology might also be used on animals (RAFI 1999).

Celia Deane-Drummond also thinks that some genetic engineering developments in wealthier countries could be devastating to certain Third World economies. For example, new means of producing vanilla and cocoa in factories in North America and/or Europe could be devastating to the economies of Madagascar and West Africa, respectively (Deane-Drummond 1995, 309). Lisa S. Cahill also thinks that genetic research and developments raise fundamental issues regarding the distribution of power and fairness. The market is a major influence in determining what research gets funded. "Discussion about genetics, ethics and social policy is now controlled almost exclusively by the academic, political and scientific elites in the First World nations of Europe and North America." She calls for a more inclusive dialogue incorporating wider global and grassroots participation since decisions about genetic practices "in fact affect the lives and futures of much larger populations" (Junker-Kenny and Cahill 1998, xii).

Catholic social teaching points out that economic activity and production are meant to provide for the needs of human beings. While this teaching acknowledges that profits are necessary to ensure the future of a business and employment, it refuses to accept the absolute primacy of the law of the marketplace over human labor. Although it also refuses to accept regulating the economy solely by centralized planning that perverts the basis for social bonds, it commends reasonable regulation of the marketplace and economic initiatives that promotes the dignity, legitimate rights and good of persons, the common good, and justice and solidarity, both within countries and internationally (CCC 1999, nn. 2419–42).

BIOLOGICAL WARFARE

Biological warfare involves using living organisms such as bacteria, viruses and fungi for military purposes. The knowledge and technology developed for commercial genetic engineering in agriculture, medicine and so forth, could potentially be used to develop a wide range of pathogens to attack plant, animal and human populations. A 1995 Central Intelligence Agency (CIA) study reported that seventeen countries, including Iraq were suspected of researching and stockpiling germ warfare agents. A number of other countries, including the United States are conducting research on biological warfare that is claimed to be defensive in nature but which is difficult to distinguish from such research for offensive purposes. The new genetic engineering technologies could provide a variety of biological warfare agents that could be developed and produced cheaply and used for a variety of military purposes. These range from terrorism, to destroying certain plants or animals to cripple a country's economy, to destroying either specific races, to large-scale warfare aimed at entire populations. Even if terrorists or military leaders do not deliberately release such agents, "the increasing experimentation with designer gene weapons in laboratories across the world…increases the likelihood of accidental releases. No laboratory, however contained and secure, is failsafe. Natural disasters such as floods and fires, and security breaches are possible and unpreventable" (Rifkin 1998, 91–96; cf. Suzuki and Knudtson 1988, Ch. 9). With regard to this issue, Pope John Paul II says, "Despite the international agreements which prohibit chemical, bacteriological and biological warfare, the fact is that laboratory research continues to develop new offensive weapons capable of altering the balance of nature" (John Paul II 1989, n. 12).

1.B. Genetically Modified Food

Some reasons raised in favor of the genetic engineering of plants and animals that result in genetically modified foods for human beings include the following: the food itself may taste better or have better nutritional value, texture and shelf life; or the plants and animals which produce the foods may yield better or be more resistant to weeds, pests and diseases requiring less use of herbicides and pesticides. Some scientists think genetically modifying certain organisms is the best way to feed adequately the approximately 800 million people who now suffer from chronic malnutrition and the three billion additional people expected to populate the earth by 2100. Without this we would need to increase significantly the use of fertilizers, herbicides and pesticides and/or to increase significantly the amount of cultivated land by converting forests and other wild lands. These would be disastrous for wildlife, result in a loss of biodiversity, and likely harm our environment (Burnett 2000; DiCenzo 2000; Reuters Feb. 29, 2000). Using genetic engineering in food production, however, raises human health and other concerns for many people.

In 1992 the Food and Drug Administration (FDA) announced that it would not require special labeling for genetically engineered foods. Critics, however, worried that introducing novel genes into common foods could cause serious allergic reactions in people. A study published in *The New England Journal of Medicine* (March 14, 1996) in fact showed that genetically engineered soybeans containing a gene from a Brazil nut could create allergic reactions in people allergic to the nut. Although the FDA says it will label genetically engineered foods containing genes from common allergenic organisms, it does not require "across-the-board" labeling. In December 1996 the European Union accepted the import of genetically modified soya bean and maize. Since these foods are used in processing many other foods, they will go untraced into many food products as well. Some think these decisions show more concern for the interests of business and winning markets than for those of ordinary people and consumers.

Many genes are being introduced into foods from plants, microorganisms and animals that have never been part of the human diet. In the coming years agrochemical and biotech companies plan to introduce hundreds of genes from other organisms including human beings into plants and animals used as human foods. The potential for serious allergic reactions in people who consume these foods is unpredictable. Some of these allergies may be life-threatening and have no known treatments.

Some argue that not requiring labeling of genetically modified foods also does not allow people of certain religions (e.g., Jews and Muslims) to know whether their food contains genes from animals (e.g., pigs) that their religion does not allow them to eat. Without labeling, vegetarians also cannot know whether or not the plants they eat contain genes from animals. Another question some ask is whether or not eating food that contained a gene or genes of human origin would be cannibalism.

In the light of such concerns regarding genetically modified foods, many are calling for laws to require the clear labeling of all such foods. Consumers would then have the right and power to choose to buy or not to buy, to eat or not to eat, these foods. In support of such a policy, a 1997 public opinion survey found that ninety-three percent of the public thought that all biotech foods should be labeled (Rifkin 1998, 103–5; SRT 1998, "Genetically Modified Food"; Wilkie 1998, 996; Bruce 1998, Ch. 6). In April 1999 Canada agreed to lead an international effort to try to reach a consensus on what labeling should be required for genetically modified foods (Bueckert 1999). The Vatican's Pontifical Academy for Life has concluded in part that the health effects of genetically altered foods "should be carefully monitored, and consumers should be informed that the foods have been altered" (Thavis 1999, 1).

1. C. Xenotransplants, Transgenic Animals and Hybrids

The demand for human organs from deceased donors for transplants far exceeds the supply. Many potential human recipients die waiting. This has spurred research into the possibility of xenotransplants, that is, transplanting an animal organ such as a liver from a baboon or a heart from a pig into a human being. In transplanting organs between human beings, unless they are identical twins, drug therapy is needed to prevent the recipient's body from rejecting the donor's organ. In transplants between species this rejection response is even more acute whereby human antibodies act rapidly to reject the transplanted tissue as though responding to an infection. Related to this, research is being carried out to try to create transgenic animals whose organs are more compatible and less likely to be rejected by human recipients. For example, research at Cambridge is attempting to transfer the appropriate human gene(s) into pigs so that their hearts are no longer recognized as foreign by human recipients.

Besides the rejection problem with xenotransplants, there may be other problems related to physiological differences such as life-span, heart rate, blood pressure and the structure of regulatory hormones between the donor animal and human recipient. Especially in the first experiments of transplants from transgenic animals it would not be possible to predict the outcome. Although the first recipients would face a very uncertain future, it is expected that some people who already face a high likelihood of death from their condition would volunteer. One of the greatest concerns with xenotransplants, however, is the possibility that the transplant might also transfer an undetected animal virus into the human being with devastating consequences (SRT 1998, "The Ethics of Xenografting").

Some viruses are harmless in one species but very harmful in another. For example, it has been discovered that a subspecies of African chimpanzee has harbored the AIDS virus for at least 100,000 years. This virus does not harm the chimpanzees but since passing over to human beings has killed many (Knox). Other viruses could possibly be transferred to humans in xenotransplants which might be harmful to human beings and transmitted to other human beings by sexual relations, and so forth, resulting in new epidemics. With regard to the risks of this, Dr. Abdallah Daar of the World Health Organization says:

> We do not have the scientific base...to assess the risks yet, we know there is a risk, we think the risk is appreciable without being able to quantify it, and we know the outcome of the risk is huge. It (the emergence of a new virus) only needs to happen once in a thousand episodes for it to be a global crisis and therefore, let's proceed with caution." (Cairney 1998)

Regulations with regard to xenotransplants are not the same in all countries. For example, they are allowed in the United States with the hope that potential benefits justify the risks. Policing experiments is left to local surgeons and institutional review boards. In the United Kingdom, however, all xenotransplants are barred "pending further study of the risks of spreading animal viruses into the human population" (Rifkin 1998, 107). The Vatican Academy for Life has said (October 1999) that the use of animal organs for transplants in humans offers potential advantages, but "such transplants should be considered morally unacceptable for the time being because of the risk of transmitting serious diseases from animals to the human species" (Thavis 1999, 5). More recently this Academy has said that animal to human transplants would be ethical "only after very strict conditions have been guaranteed" (Zenit Sept. 26, 2001).

Animal suffering is another issue that experiments in developing transgenic animals raises. Such research is being conducted on thousands of animals from mice to livestock to primates in the attempt to find cures for certain human diseases, to improve livestock, and so forth. Introducing foreign genes into the genetic code of an animal, however, often produces multiple and unpredictable reactions, sometimes causing animals unprecedented suffering. A few actual examples follow of such experiments that have resulted in animals with more stress, serious health problems and/or serious abnormalities. In one experiment a transgene composed of a gene from a fruit fly and another from a virus was inserted into mouse embryos. Some of the newborn mice had extreme abnormalities including loss of hind limbs, facial clefts and massive brain defects. In another experiment a human growth hormone gene was introduced into pig embryos, hoping to produce larger, faster-growing pigs. Unexpectedly, the resultant pigs included ones with arthritis, degenerating muscles and other gross abnormalities. Posilac, a genetically engineered drug designed to increase milk production in cows by as much as twenty percent, is currently marketed in the

United States by Monsanto. Many dairy farmers who have tried this drug, however, have experienced a host of health problems, and an increase of stress and death in their herds (Rifkin 1998, 96–99).

With regard to using animals in research, many call for showing proper respect to the animals and minimizing their pain, including the use of pain relief (e.g., Roy et al. 1994, 333; and CHAC 2000, 66). The Vatican's Pontifical Academy for Life has concluded that although it can be licit to genetically modify animals in order to improve human health and living conditions, it is not acceptable to cause suffering to an animal without a reason "proportional to its social usefulness" (Thavis 1999, 1; cf. Bruce 1998, Ch. 5).

Concerning religious perspectives on these issues, we can note, for example, that the Hebrew Bible (the Old Testament) forbids the cross breeding of distinct plant and animal "kinds" (Lev 19:19). It also forbids humans from having sexual relations with animals (Lev 18:23). In the light of this, some Christians, Jews and Muslims might argue that we should not make transgenic plants and animals or intermingle the human and animal with xenotransplants. The distinction of "kinds" reflects the goodness, purposes and wisdom of the Creator. Radically altering the created order might be seen by some as proud human beings not properly respecting God the Creator and his created order. Some others, however, would argue that our technology and medicine already alter the created order in radical ways. Why draw the line here, that is, at xenotransplants and transgenic animals? The normal Christian understanding believes Jesus Christ has fulfilled and superceded the numerous ceremonial regulations in the Old Testament, such as which animals may be eaten (cf. Acts 10). In the light of this, some Christians would not object to xenotransplants and transgenic animals in principle (SRT 1998, "The Ethics of Xenografting").

Perhaps a more radical mixing of "kinds" than introducing one or even a few foreign genes into an animal embryo to make a transgenic animal is producing an animal hybrid. Since the 1960s scientists have succeeded in producing hybrid cell cultures, plants and animals by artificially fusing certain cells. Some of these, such as producing hybrid cell cultures to produce large numbers of identical antibodies, could have some useful purposes. With regard to animals, experiments fusing two early embryos or mixing totipotent cells from two embryos have resulted in mice, rabbits and sheep, and the like, who have not two but four parents. The resultant chimera is actually a "mosaic" having two different genetic types. Some organs or parts of organs are from one set of parents and other organs or parts of organs are from the other set of parents. Using this technique scientists have also succeeded in producing hybrid animals from two different species such as a half sheep and half goat or "geep." It is speculated that it may be possible to make an animal/human hybrid in this way, such as a chimp/hume, half chimpanzee and half human. Such animal/human chimeras could perhaps be used in medical research and/or as potential organ donors (Varga 1984, 115–16; and Rifkin 1998, 2–3 and 101).

Canada's Royal Commission on New Reproductive Technologies "recommends that some current and potential practices are so harmful and so sharply contravene Canadian ethical and social values that they should not be permitted in Canada on threat of criminal sanction. These include research involving...creation of animal/human hybrids..." (RCNRT 1993, 5; cf. Bill C-47 1996; and MRCC et al. 1998, 9.3). Andrew Varga thinks that using cell fusion to make new species of plants or animals may have some useful purposes but care would need to be taken to prevent such organisms from getting out of control and causing great harm. He thinks that making an animal/human hybrid, however, would be unethical and such experiments should not be attempted. This would not elevate animals but degrade and dehumanize human beings (Varga 1984, 123–24). The Vatican's Congregation for the Doctrine of the Faith also teaches that "forms of biological and genetic manipulation of human embryos, such as attempts or plans for fertilization between human and animal gametes and the gestation of human embryos in the uterus of animals...are contrary to the human dignity proper to the embryo, and at the same time they are contrary to the right of every person to be conceived and to be born within marriage and from marriage" (CDF 1987, I.6).

1.D. Cloning Plants and Animals

News in February 1997 of the cloned sheep Dolly, which seemed to bring the possibility of human cloning much closer than previously thought, provoked worldwide debate. In this section we will focus on the issue of cloning plants and animals (the issue of cloning human beings will be treated below in Ch. 2 E). Many lower forms of life produce asexually. Their offspring is a genetically similar clone. Higher plants and animals reproduce sexually by the union of germ cells. The offspring is genetically different from both parents. Nevertheless, since ancient times people have produced many genetically similar plants by cutting and planting a slip. In very early animal embryos all or some of the cells are totipotent or undifferentiated. If such embryos are split, naturally or artificially, identical twins or triplets, and so on, may be produced. These are genetically similar clones. Before Dolly, scientists had also succeeded in cloning some animals (e.g., frogs and mice) by removing the nuclei from either fertilized or unfertilized eggs and replacing them with nuclei of undifferentiated cells from other embryos. They had also succeeded in cloning some non–mammal adult vertebrates (e.g., a toad) by replacing the nucleus in the egg with the nucleus from a somatic cell of the adult (Varga 1984, 119–22; Flaman 2001, 3–4).

Before Dolly many considered the somatic cell nuclear transfer cloning of an adult mammal to be some time away or perhaps even impossible. Unlike undifferentiated cells in the early embryo which can give rise to any cell in the body, somatic adult cells are differentiated to form skin, muscle, brain, and so forth. Although all somatic cells in an individual contain the same DNA (unless mutations have occurred), almost all of the genes except for the gene(s) needed to perform the required specialized function in the differentiated cell are permanently turned off. In producing Dolly, Dr. Ian Wilmut and his team at the Roslin Institute near Edinburgh, Scotland, placed mammary cells from an adult sheep in a culture and starved them of nutrients for several days. It is believed that few if any genes remained switched on. The scientists then performed nuclear transfer 277 times, removing a nucleus from an egg cell and replacing it with a nucleus taken out of one of the mammary cells (an electric current was used to fuse the donor nucleus with the enuculated egg cell), again and again. Although the precise mechanism is not completely understood, the egg cells were able to reprogram the donor nuclei to behave as if they had come from undifferentiated cells. Any embryos that resulted were implanted into surrogates. Dolly was the only lamb to be born. In this type of cloning, the clone has the same nuclear DNA as the original adult animal, but there are some differences in the DNA in the mitochondria since these were not replaced in the egg cell (Klotzko 1997, 427–28). In 1998 scientists in Japan cloned several calves from a single adult cow (Weiss 1998). Some other species including mice and pigs have also been cloned. Although some of these cloned animals appear to be normal, others have developed various problems such as tumors, obesity, and heart, blood, lung or liver problems. Some have died prematurely. Some cloned animals develop normally for a time, even to adulthood, and then develop serious problems. Evidence seems to indicate that the rapid reprogramming that takes place during the cloning process often results in random errors in the clone's DNA. These errors can produce unpredictable problems for which we have no known methods to detect. At present animal cloning works in less than two percent of cases. Researchers in this area emphasize that this technology is still "new and unsafe" (Rogers 2000; BioNews Mar. 12, 2001, "Reproductive Cloning Isn't Safe").

Although somatic cell nuclear transfer cloning at present is very limited in its use (Wevrick 1999), developing cloning technologies are expected to make possible the mass production of identical or nearly identical copies of a plant or animal with certain desirable traits. This could include cloning transgenic plants or animals such as animals genetically engineered to produce a range of drugs and medicines in their milk or for xenotransplant purposes. If the previously mentioned problems could be overcome, cloning would enable a degree of quality control and predictability not possible with normal heterosexual reproduction (Rifkin 1998, 20–21; Klotzko 1997, 428). Some speculate that cloning technologies may also make it possible to bring back into existence certain extinct species. With regard to this, some scientists are already attempting to bring back a number of extinct species, for example, the mammoth, by defrosting living cells from frozen carcasses found in Siberia, and transferring their nuclei into enucleated elephant eggs (see Varga 1984, 122; Kotulak 1997; and Hellen 2000). Using somewhat similar ideas, the *Jurassic Park* movies cinematically recreate a number of long extinct dinosaur species.

A growing number of scientists and others are worried about the loss of genetic diversity on the earth. Major causes of this are the extinction of many species and many varieties within species. Large-scale monoculturing in agriculture, that is, large-scale production of one or only a few varieties of certain crops and herds, has contributed to the latter. Critics worry that large-scale cloning of a few varieties could lead to further reduction in genetic diversity. While mass production of certain plants and animals with a special trait or traits, by means of cloning and monoculturing, may have certain commercial and human advantages, such plants and animals could be more vulnerable to disease and super bugs. With regard to this consider, for example, the Irish potato famine in the 1840s which resulted in over a million people dying. This famine was the result of growing a genetically limited stock of potato (compare monoculturing) which turned out to be highly vulnerable to a blight which attacked the potato crop for five years (Rifkin 1998, 107–15).

A 1997 report of the Society, Religion and Technology Project of the Church of Scotland speaks too of a need to maintain the genetic diversity of animals. Nevertheless, it concludes that limited cloning of animals could be ethical, for example, if it were necessary to clone five to ten animals from a single genetically modified animal to begin a herd. These animals could then be bred naturally to give flocks of varied sheep, but all containing the desired genetic modification, such as sheep that produce a therapeutic protein in their milk for cystic fibrosis sufferers. Once past the experimental stage, such genetic engineering of animals and limited cloning of them could result in clear human benefits with few animal welfare and other concerns. This report, however, concludes that routine cloning of animals where natural methods of reproducing animals exist would bring mass production principles of the factory too far into the animal kingdom (SRT 1998, "Cloning Animals and Humans"; cf. Bruce 1998, Ch. 2.11).

A 1989 statement by the German Catholic bishops states that the variety of plant and animal species is a worldwide patrimony that must be safeguarded. Bishop Elio Sgreccia, the Vatican's leading expert on medical ethics, says there is a duty to protect various animal species from arbitrary genetic alterations. Animal cloning should be performed only under strict ethical guidelines, maintaining respect of various species. Those who see plants and animals only in terms of utility misunderstand the true value of creation. Fr. Mark Miller, director of the Redemptorist Bioethical Consultancy for Western Canada, also concludes that some cloning of animals may be justified, but warns that market forces could lead to a misuse of the technology without proper ethical considerations (Gonzalez 1997).

1.E. Patenting Life Forms

Patent law was developed originally in an industrial context to prevent unfair exploitation of human inventions. One could not patent a mere discovery. There had to be a novel, non-obvious "inventive step" and some specified practical application. In 1971

Chakrabarty, a microbiologist, applied to the U.S. Patents and Trademark Office (PTO) for a genetically engineered microorganism designed to consume oil spills on the oceans. The PTO rejected the request arguing that living things can not be patented. This was appealed and won—a narrow majority of the court ruled that the fact that the microorganisms are alive is without legal significance. This was again appealed to the U.S. Supreme Court, which ruled in 1980 (five to four) in favor of Chakrabarty, granting a patent on the first genetically engineered life form. The majority of the court argued that the relevant distinction was not between living and inanimate things, but whether or not the microbe was a "human-made invention." In 1987 the PTO ruled that all genetically engineered multicellular living organisms, including animals, are potentially patentable. This includes the possibility of patenting even parts of humans such as genetically altered genes, cell lines and organs, but does not include patenting a whole human being. The latter was seen as analogous to human slavery. Although previous patent rulings excluded claiming discoveries of nature as inventions, the PTO also said that isolating and classifying a gene's properties and purposes is sufficient to claim it as an invention. A year later, the PTO granted a patent on a mammal, a genetically engineered mouse with human genes predisposing it to develop cancer. Since then several other genetically engineered animals have been patented and many others are awaiting approval. Today there is "fierce competition between chemical, pharmaceutical, agribusiness, and biotech companies for commercial patents on genes, organisms, and processes to manipulate them...." There are also a record number of legal challenges in the United States and Europe related to charges of "patent infringements, unfair use of prior art, stealing of trade secrets, and pirating of research...as companies jostle with each other to improve their market share and competitive position" (Rifkin 1998, 41–48; cf. SRT 1998, "Patenting Life?").

Some Third World countries are also seeking compensation, a portion of the gains from patented products, from transnational biotech companies. Such companies they claim are often getting a "free ride," merely isolating, slightly engineering and patenting products that indigenous peoples, villagers and farmers have developed over centuries, by isolating, enhancing and preserving valuable herbs and plant crops. Despite their differences, both these companies and Third World countries are regarding the global gene pool as a commodity that can be priced in the marketplace. Another position being advanced by some non-governmental organizations and countries is that "the gene pool ought not to be for sale, at any price—that it should remain an open commons and continue to be used freely by present and future generations." Compare the continent of Antarctica which has been kept "as a global commons free of commercial exploitation" (Rifkin 1998, 48–55).

The issue of patenting life forms has become very controversial. On the one hand, much of the biotechnological industry argues that without patent protection no one will invest the large sums of money required for genetic research or the information will not be shared. Breakthroughs in this area, including the development of genetically altered life forms with desirable traits and therapeutic products, often follow years of expensive research. Copying the results of such expensive research, however, is often much easier and less expensive. If life forms cannot be patented it is argued by many that many potential benefits to human beings will be lost, including the development of some new cures or treatments for certain human cancers and other diseases. Avoidable suffering will go unalleviated. Or, economic opportunities will be lost to other nations who are not as restrictive.

On the other hand many, including a number of non-governmental organizations, ecological groups, animal rights activists, indigenous peoples, and religious groups have expressed opposition or grave concerns regarding patenting life. For some, patenting life forms implies that living organisms are nothing more than machines, products of manufacture, and are only seen in terms of their utility to us rather than as God's creatures having inherent

worth. Some argue that living organisms and their genes are products of nature or created by God and so cannot be claimed as
human inventions (SRT 1998, "Patenting Life?"; cf. Walter 2000,
132–33; and Kaveny 1999, 146). Some critics also argue that "the
commercially driven nature of biotech research has seriously
undermined the traditional collegial laboratory atmosphere of
sharing ideas and has slowed cooperative efforts to find solutions to
problems. Secrecy has become paramount in a commercially
directed system where the reward for research is no longer simply
the respect and admiration of peers and contribution to knowledge
but rather the patenting of potentially lucrative inventions" (Rifkin
1998, 56).

A 1995 Declaration of Indigenous Peoples of the Western
Hemisphere states in part: "We oppose the patenting of all natural
genetic materials. We hold that life cannot be bought, owned, sold,
discovered or patented, even in its smallest form" (Indigenous
Peoples 1995).

In May 1995, a coalition of more than 200 U.S. religious leaders,
including more than 100 Catholic bishops; leaders from virtually
every major Protestant denomination; and Jewish, Muslim, Bud-
dhist and Hindu leaders announced their opposition "to the granting of patents on animal and human genes, organs, tissues, and
organisms." Although all these religious leaders did not oppose
"process" patents "for the techniques used to create transgenic life
forms, they were unanimous in their opposition to the patenting of
the life forms and the parts themselves. They were keenly aware of
the profound consequences of shifting authorship from God to scientists and transnational companies..." (Rifkin 1998, 65–66). The
Vatican's Pontifical Academy for Life has said in part (October
1999) that "when patents are given, a distinction should be made
between what is found in nature and what is specifically designed
for commercial sale....The human genetic code, human embryos
and human cloning procedures should never be patented" (Thavis
1999, 1 and 5; cf. CHAC 2000, 65).

The Society, Religion and Technology Project of the Church of Scotland suggests that we perhaps need a new system of intellectual property involving living material instead of shoring up a patenting system that was not designed to handle such cases. While there is a good case, for example, of a pharmaceutical company gaining a patent to use a gene sequence to produce a particular therapeutic drug, many see it as claiming too much to seek a patent on the sequence itself for any use whatsoever by virtue of having invested a lot of money in isolating it and identifying its function. Such could hamper research by preventing other companies from investing in other therapeutic uses of the same gene. This project recommends that a statutory national ethical commission be set up whereby biotechnological inventions can be made public, and given interim intellectual property protection, while the public is granted opportunity to voice objections or support and to appeal. "If something is not done to grant such a public debate, the controversy over patenting living organisms will continue without any hope of resolution, and, in the long run, the bioindustry risks losing part of its public for the wrong reasons" (SRT 1998, "Patenting Life?"; cf. Bruce 1998, Ch. 8).

Discussion Questions

1. What, if any, are some of the real and potential benefits of genetically engineering some plants and animals? Do you think the genetic engineering of some plants and animals is necessary to feed the growing human population? What risks do these entail for the environment and human beings? Should all genetically modified food products be labeled? Why do you think that some governments do not require the clear labeling of all genetically modified foods? (See Chs. 1.A and 1.B above).

2. How would you feel about receiving a heart from a genetically modified pig or chimpanzee? What are the possible benefits and risks of xenotransplants? (See Ch. 1.C above).

3. Do you think there should be any legal regulations regarding genetically modified organisms (GMOs), the genetic engineering of plants and animals? If so, what laws should we have? What are the reasons for your position? If you were a scientist working in these areas, would participating in any types of research (e.g., regarding biological warfare or research that causes some animals to suffer) be against your conscience? What do you think of patenting life forms? (See Ch. 1 above.)

Chapter Two

Genetic Engineering of Human Beings

In this chapter we will consider a number of ethical issues related to the genetic engineering of human beings. This includes both engineering certain genetic traits into human individuals and the human gene pool as well as means of attempting to get rid of or engineering certain genetic traits out of existence.

2.A. Genetic Testing and Screening

The number of people with a genetic disorder or disease should not be exaggerated. Most human babies are born healthy and many people are healthy for much of their lives. Even so-called "normal" people generally experience some illnesses in life and some debilitating conditions before they die. Such facts should be kept in mind to keep the whole area of genetic testing and screening in proper perspective. That being said, we can note, for example, that it is estimated that there are about 4,000 human diseases that are inherited or related to genetic factors. At present, genetic centers in North America offer tests for some thirty to forty of the more commonly inherited disorders including cystic fibrosis, Huntington's disease, Duchenne muscular dystrophy, susceptibility to some types of breast cancer, and various types of degeneration of the brainstem, spinal cord and peripheral nerves. If one includes variants of some diseases, the number of DNA probes available is around 400 with the number increasing (Golden 1999, 40–42. For information on specific inherited disorders see GeneClinics). Genetic tests can be carried out at various stages in an individual's life including before birth, before the embryo is implanted, and after birth, including before a person gets married or conceives a child.

(1) PRENATAL DIAGNOSIS, FETAL THERAPY AND ABORTION

There are several methods of prenatal diagnosis—tests before birth to determine whether or not the fetus is "normal" or "abnormal" in some way. Amniocentesis has been used since the 1950s. It involves analyzing fetal cells obtained from amniotic fluid samples obtained by needle aspiration under ultrasound guidance. Amniocentesis is often performed around the sixteenth week of pregnancy. There is some risk of miscarriage as a result of amniocentesis—less than one percent with the help of sonography (Ashley and O'Rourke 1997, 250). Chorionic villus sampling has been used clinically since 1984. It analyzes bits of chorionic villi that surround the amniotic sac and that contain the chromosomes and genes of the fetus. This method can be performed between eight and nine weeks of pregnancy, often enabling a woman to request an abortion before her family or friends realize she is pregnant. It carries a higher risk of miscarriages of normal fetuses than amniocentesis, however, and may cause malformations, such as limb malformations in otherwise healthy fetuses. Whether it causes malformations is at present controversial, not proven fact (Wevrick 1999). Ultrasound, which is now used routinely to monitor pregnancies in many countries, can provide reliable diagnosis of a wide range of fetal abnormalities with expert interpretation. Maternal serum alpha-fetoprotein screening has been available since the 1980s. High levels of alpha-fetoprotein in a pregnant woman's blood may indicate that the fetus has a neural tube defect, for example, anencephaly or spina bifida. It may produce false positive results, implying that the fetus has a certain defect when in fact it is healthy, causing anxiety until another test shows the fetus to be unaffected (Roy et al. 1994, 178–79). It should be noted that there is also some chance of false positives with the other prenatal tests, since no such test is 100 percent reliable. The results of amniocentesis and chorionic villus sampling may also be confused by so-called chromosomal structural abnormalities, which may or may not have a genetically significant effect. Although some genetic tests are among the most accurate of medical tests considered in the context of all of medicine (Wevrick 1999), not all prenatal tests provide the clear-cut answers that some would like (Golden 1999, 40).

The goals of prenatal diagnosis vary. They include: (1) to have a normal child, using selective abortion if there is a positive diagnosis; (2) to give parents information they can use to better prepare themselves to care for a disabled child; (3) to prevent, treat and/or cure fetal problems diagnosed before birth (today many such problems diagnosed before birth cannot be treated, but with advancing fetal and gene therapy, the therapeutic goal may become more achievable); and (4) to control the quality of the population. Although this last goal may not be a widespread political goal today, prenatal diagnosis programs and the choice of many parents to use selective abortion can lead to significant reductions in the birth rates of babies with various kinds of genetic disorders (Roy et al. 1994, 180–81). For example, prenatal screening and selective abortions have reduced by "more than 95% the number of Tay-Sachs births among American Jews of East European descent, a high-risk group"(Golden 1999, 42).

FETAL THERAPY

Fetal Therapy began in the early 1960s when "Dr. Liley successfully administered intrauterine blood transfusions to fetuses who, otherwise, would have died from severe anemia resulting from rhesus incompatibility with the mother" (Roy et al. 1994, 183). Although many disorders diagnosed prenatally cannot be treated, there are already several options that may be beneficial regarding a number of conditions. In some cases, advancing the time of delivery can permit early treatment of some conditions that otherwise would cause severe harm or death to the fetus. Cesarian delivery can be used in cases where vaginal delivery would threaten the child or mother. In some cases, prenatal diagnosis can assist in preparing for immediate treatment after birth. There has also been some success in treating fetuses with some conditions before birth with surgery (e.g., hydrocephaly and certain heart problems), with experimental surgery (e.g., spina bifida), or with drugs (e.g., adrenal hyperplasia). It is interesting to note that this branch of medicine considers the fetus a patient distinct from the mother.

Recent studies demonstrate that there is a certain time during development, estimated between twelve and fourteen weeks, during which the human fetus cannot immunologically reject foreign tissue. Therapeutic transplants of tissues or cells to the fetus during this time would thus not be expected to pose the difficulties due to tissue incompatibility of postnatal (after birth) transplants. The Food and Drug Administration (FDA) has already received several requests to use bone marrow cells to treat fetuses in utero. The goals of such transplantation would include: "(1) establishing normal cellular function before the target organ damage occurs; (2) establishing stable and durable chimerism that will obviate or diminish the need for post natal transplants; and (3) inducing donor-specific tolerance that would permit post-natal transplants with minimal or no preparative immunosuppression" (Frank Young in Kilner et al. 1997, 177).

Since interventions regarding the fetus also involve interventions on the woman, her free and informed consent is required (MRCC et al. 1998, 9.5). There have been legal court cases where invasive medical interventions on an adult against his or her clear wishes, expressed while considered legally competent, have been deemed a form of assault or battery. From an ethical perspective, one would need to consider whether or not the expected benefit to the fetus is proportionate to any risks or harm to the mother (Roy et al. 1994, 183–87; cf. Shannon 2000, 112). From a Catholic perspective, one has a moral obligation to consent to "ordinary" medical treatments, that is, treatments which offer a reasonable hope of proportionate benefit, without grave burdens for the patient or others. One is not obliged to use "extraordinary" treatments, however, which are disproportionate or which involve grave burdens for the patient or others. This would also apply to a guardian or proxy who should act in the best interests of an incompetent person, taking into account any known and reasonable wishes he or she may have expressed (see, e.g., USCC 1994, nn. 23–28 and 55–59; and CHAC 2000, 13–14, 32 and 56–59). Concerning this and fetal therapy, consider the pregnant woman on behalf of the child within her, as well as the proxy of an incompetent pregnant woman.

Canada's Royal Commission on New Reproductive Technologies says that there is "a great deal of misinformation" about prenatal diagnosis. Among other things, this Commission concluded that "there is a need for accurate, unbiased, accessible information in this field. It is important that all eligible women be informed of the service and that their wishes to use or not use the technology be respected"; prenatal testing that is "unable to provide useful or reliable information about the likelihood of a person becoming ill…would not be an effective or responsible investment of scarce health care resources"; and "sex-selective abortion, simply because one sex is preferred over the other, is…incompatible with Canadian values. It violates the principles of respect for human life and dignity, protection of the vulnerable, and appropriate use of resources"

(RCNRT 1993, 15–16). Sex-selective abortions have been done not only in places of the world, such as China and India, where many prefer to have a boy rather than a girl, but also elsewhere "as a means of ensuring sibling gender balance" in families (Rifkin 1998, 140).

ABORTION

Based on scientific evidence and sound reasoning, Catholic teaching concludes that not only the human fetus, but also the human embryo and zygote, is already a human being. It has its own genetic program and is an individual distinct from both its mother and father. Based on this conclusion, Catholic teaching has defended the basic rights, in particular the right to life, of the human zygote, embryo and fetus. With regard to this, the Vatican's Congregation for the Doctrine of the Faith teaches in part that

> the fruit of human generation, from the first moment of its existence, that is to say from the moment the zygote has formed, demands the unconditional respect that is morally due to the human being in his bodily and spiritual totality. The human being is to be respected and treated as a person from the moment of conception; and therefore from that same moment his rights as a person must be recognized, among which in the first place is the inviolable right of every innocent human being to life. (CDF 1987, I.1)

Pope John Paul II in *The Gospel of Life,* teaches that "*direct abortion, that is, abortion willed as an end or as a means, always constitutes a grave moral disorder,* since it is the deliberate killing of an innocent human being" (John Paul II, 1995b, n. 62). Among other things, he speaks sympathetically to women who have had an abortion, addressing their need for healing. He says in part, "...do not lose hope....If you have not already done so, give yourselves over with humility and trust to repentance. The Father of mercies is ready to give you his forgiveness and his peace..." (John Paul II, 1995b, n.

99; see also Linn and Fabricant 1985). With regard to prenatal diagnosis in the same document Pope John Paul II says:

> Special attention must be given to evaluating the morality of *prenatal diagnostic techniques* which enable the early detection of possible anomalies in the unborn child. In view of the complexity of these techniques, an accurate and systematic moral judgment is necessary. When they do not involve disproportionate risks for the child and the mother, and are meant to make possible early therapy or even to favor a serene and informed acceptance of the child not yet born, these techniques are morally licit. But since the possibilities of prenatal therapy are still limited, it not infrequently happens that these techniques are used with a eugenic intention which accepts selective abortion in order to prevent the birth of children affected by various types of anomalies. Such an attitude is shameful and utterly reprehensible, since it presumes to measure the value of a human life only within the parameters of "normality" and physical well-being, thus opening the way to legitimizing infanticide and euthanasia as well.
>
> And yet the courage and the serenity with which so many of our brothers and sisters suffering from serious disabilities lead their lives when they are shown acceptance and love bears eloquent witness to what gives authentic value to life, and makes it, even in difficult conditions, something precious for them and for others. The Church is close to those married couples who with great anguish and suffering, willingly accept gravely handicapped children. She is also grateful to all those families which, through adoption, welcome children abandoned by their parents because of disabilities or illnesses. (John Paul II 1995b, n. 63; cf. CDF 1987, I.2–3; USCC 1994, n. 50, and 1996; CHAUSA 1990; and Thavis 1999, 5)

With regard to prenatal diagnosis and the possibility of "false positives," William May says that advocating abortion in these cases includes a willingness to kill unborn children who are not suffering from any genetic defect. Calling such abortion "therapeutic" is a misuse of language since it is hardly therapeutic for the fetus. Anyone choosing direct abortion (the direct object of one's act is to kill the human fetus or unborn child), for any reason, takes on the moral identity of a killer and sets one's heart against a fellow human being (May 1977, 89–90 and 104–5; see also May 2000, Ch. 5).

For a fuller treatment of the question "When Does Human Life Begin?" and abortion, including lifesaving treatments of the mother and "indirect" abortion, see, for example, Benedict Ashley and Kevin O'Rourke 1997, Ch. 9.1 and Ch. 9.4, respectively. The videos, "Who Should Decide? Prenatal Diagnosis" (NFB 1986) and "On the Eighth Day: Perfecting Mother Nature" (CBC 1992), both treat the issues of prenatal diagnosis, selective abortion and human disabilities. The latter video includes interviews with several disabled people who have a high appreciation of the value of their own lives.

Concerning these issues Ben Mitchell asks us to "imagine, if Dr. Hawking's parents had had access to prenatal genetic screening technology." Dr. Steven Hawking, a renowned physicist, has been suffering from a genetic illness, Lou Gehrig's disease, for over twenty years (Kilner et al. 1997, 242–43). It is also worth noting, for example, that Jean Vanier's L'Arche communities, talks and books demonstrate a profound appreciation for the value of the lives of disabled people. Eduardo Rodriguez counters those who favor selective abortion to prevent suffering, saying that

> there is no life without some kind of suffering and therefore the elimination of suffering can not be the basis for not allowing somebody to develop. At the same time, society has the duty to try to provide the best environment possible to diminish the suffering of individuals born with diseases, thus exercising compassion and care, which forms human character and gives a value to the suffering of those individuals. (Rodriguez 2000, 35)

(2) PREIMPLANTATION GENETIC DIAGNOSIS

Preimplantation Genetic Diagnosis (PGD) has been used to test for a number of genetic diseases, such as hemophilia, Duchenne muscular dystrophy and cystic fibrosis, since 1993. PGD involves removing a cell from a preimplantation embryo in vitro and analyzing its DNA. By a method called polymerase chain reaction, the amount of DNA extracted from even one embryonic cell can be quickly increased so that there is enough for diagnosis. Since there are both mild and severe forms of diseases such as cystic fibrosis, preimplantation tests may not give a clear prognosis of how severely affected the child will be. Nevertheless, with in vitro fertilization (IVF) and PGD only those embryos that pass the "test" are candidates to be transferred into the uterus of a woman. Generally a few "normal" embryos are transferred with the hopes that one or more will implant and develop into a baby. Embryos which do not pass the test may be experimented on and are discarded. IVF with PGD thus involves both positive and negative eugenics—choosing embryonic human beings with "normal" or desirable genetic characteristics to continue living and destroying those embryonic human beings with "unwanted" genetic characteristics. While abortion is often a painful decision, many people find it to be a lot less of a problem to not implant and discard some "sixteen-cell embryos." Both IVF and PGD are expensive procedures. IVF and embryo transfer costs several thousand dollars per attempt. With its low success rate many couples spend tens of thousands of dollars before having a baby or perhaps not having one at all. PGD costs $20,000 to screen for a single disease. Since these costs are prohibitive for most couples, PGD is very rarely done (CBC 1992; Roy et al. 1994, 182–83; Golden 1999, 42; and Wevrick 1999).

Examination of the human zygote or preimplantation embryonic human being can reveal his or her sex. With regard to this, Canada's Royal Commission on New Reproductive Technologies concluded that "sex-selective zygote transfer...simply because of a preference" is inappropriate for the same reasons as sex-selective abortion (see under 2.A.1 above; RCNRT 1993, 16). Both this Royal Commission and the Medical Research Council of Canada would allow non-therapeutic research on spare embryos and discarding of embryos up to fourteen days, at which point the embryo starts to develop the primitive streak, the first indication of neural development. They, however, oppose creating human embryos simply for research purposes (RCNRT 1993, 14; and MRCC et al. 1998, 9.4).

In the United States no federal research funds may be used for the creation of a human embryo for research purposes or for research in which a human embryo is destroyed, discarded or knowingly subjected to more than minimal risk (see NIH 1997, "Directives on Human Embryo Research." Cf. Kaveny 1999, 137; and 2.E.2 below regarding "Cloning Human Embryos for 'Therapeutic' Purposes").

Catholic teaching, based on scientific evidence and sound reasoning, affirms that the human zygote and embryo already is a human being to be respected as a person (see 2.A.1 above). Discarding or destroying human zygotes and embryos, which is normally associated with in vitro fertilization (IVF), is thus morally equivalent to abortion. The Vatican's Congregation for the Doctrine of the Faith also considers IVF to violate the rights of the child to be conceived within his or her mother as a fruit of a conjugal act, a reciprocal act of self-giving love between spouses. As well, IVF "establishes the domination of technology over the origin and destiny of the human person. Such a relationship of domination is in itself contrary to the dignity and equality that must be common to parents and children" (CDF 1987, II.1–5). This Congregation considers research on the human embryo licit that only involves observation and poses no risks to it. It also says that therapeutic research that aims to benefit the embryo, as a final attempt to save its life and in the absence of other reliable forms of therapy, can be licit. It, however, regards illicit all invasive experimentation on human embryos that is not directly therapeutic and that always involves risks to its integrity or life (CDF

1987, I.4). The Vatican's Pontifical Academy for Life has said (October 1999) that, "...genetic diagnosis of embryos before implantation in the womb is immoral, because it represents a selective method that results in the destruction of 'sick' embryos, and in general is used along with in vitro fertilization, which is rejected by Church teaching" (Thavis 1999, 5; cf. May 2000, Ch. 6.5.B).

Although preimplantation genetic tests would need to become considerably less expensive for them to be used widely, prenatal and preimplantation genetic tests are likely to increase as more tests become available. It is also likely that there will be growing pressures on doctors and parents to be "genetically responsible" by having genetic tests. In the United States there have already been a few hundred ominous "wrongful birth" and/or "wrongful life" lawsuits. In these, parents have attempted to sue physicians for not making available information on screening procedures that could have been performed and whose results could have been used by them to decide whether or not to abort the fetus (Rifkin 1998 138–39). Also very disturbing are statements such as "individuals have a paramount right to be born with a normal, adequate hereditary endowment" made by the United State's Congressional Office of Technology Assessment (cited in Asch and Geller 1996, 323). While increased genetic knowledge may empower some people, many people, including some feminists, are concerned that it may also reduce some women's choices or support if the larger society believes they could have avoided certain problems by testing (Asch and Geller 1996, 325).

From the end of the Second World War through the 1980s, social scientists and politicians generally favored nurture over nature with regard to addressing social evils. In recent years scientists have been finding more links between behavior, personality and genetics. Although sociobiologists still acknowledge that environment plays a role in individual and group development, there is now often more emphasis on the role genes play, that is, more emphasis on nature. Today more people are arguing that genes are at the root of many social problems. New experimental research by developmental geneticists, however, is undermining assumptions based on simple genetic reductionism and may help provide a much needed balance in understanding "the many subtle relationships that exist between genotype and phenotype [the observable characteristics of an organism or group] and between environmental triggers and genetic expression." The focus on genetics alone as explanatory of disease and social problems shifts society's attention away from other means of dealing with such problems (Rifkin 1998, Ch. 5; the quotation is from 156). Many people, including some feminists, are concerned that narrow views of biological reductionism could result in less funding for social solutions to human problems (Asch and Geller 1996, 326–27).

(3) GENETIC TESTING AFTER BIRTH

Most postnatal genetic tests are physically harmless, only involving the withdrawal of an insignificant amount of body fluid or tissue (Ashley and O'Rourke 1997, 325). In many places genetic screening of all newborns for phenylketonuria (PKU) is mandatory. This test is quite inexpensive. Individuals with PKU have a metabolic disorder and lack the enzyme necessary to convert the amino acid phenylalanine into tyrosine. Accumulation of phenylalanine is toxic to brain tissue. Among other things, untreated individuals suffer from progressive mental retardation. Treatment for individuals with PKU consists of a diet free of phenylalanine (Urdang et al. 1983, 839). Since the benefits of this program of genetic screening clearly seem to outweigh the drawbacks, few have objected to this.

This has not been the case, however, with all attempts to genetically screen a certain population. For example, in the 1970s in a number of U.S. states mass genetic-screening laws for sickle-cell anemia created great confusion, anxiety and a hostile response in the black population. Most black legislators originally strongly supported these laws that have since been repealed. Sickle-cell anemia is a painful crippling disease that leads to early death and affects black persons almost exclusively. Attempts by companies to screen their workers for genetic predispositions to certain illnesses that might be triggered by materials used in the workplace, or by insurance companies to screen prospective clients, have also raised serious concerns regarding discrimination. Andrew Varga concludes that any mass genetic screening "should be limited to genetic defects that can be diagnosed with certitude and are greatly debilitating. The public should be adequately informed and educated...in order to avoid misunderstandings and stigmatization." They should be accessible to everybody and generally voluntary (Varga 1984, 84–87; cf. Bryannan 1999; and Rodriguez 2000, 29 and 35). The widely accepted principle of free and informed consent would require that any genetic testing of competent adults be both voluntary and informed. Even with incompetent subjects such as young children, the wishes of guardians should be respected unless such would result in serious harm to the incompetent subjects that can be clearly prevented. Guardians should act in the best interests of incompetent subjects, taking into account their reasonable wishes if they have or can express their wishes (cf. Ashley and O'Rourke 1997, 186–87 and 325–27).

Huntington's disease is a rare hereditary condition that causes progressively serious mental and physical disabilities and then death later in life. The first signs usually show up between thirty and forty-five years of age, and the person dies about fifteen years later. At present there is no treatment. If one has a parent with Huntington's disease, one has a fifty percent chance of having it. There now exists a genetic test by means of which a presymptomatic individual can find out whether or not he or she will develop the symptoms later in life. More and more genetic tests after birth are being developed for other conditions that one may develop later in life or have a predisposition for such as breast cancer, diabetes and cardiovascular disease. For some of these, altering one's diet and lifestyle may reduce one's chances of developing the disease if one has the predisposing gene or genes (cf. Roy et al. 1994, 451–52).

Some forms of postnatal genetic testing are already reaping incredible health benefits. For example, genetic testing for cystic fibrosis, which has largely replaced the sweat test in infants and young children, "has allowed early treatment and improved prognosis in those affected with the disease. Another example is hemachromatosis, a disease of iron storage that affects one in 300 people of Northern European descent. If untreated, it causes liver cancer and diabetes; treatment to remove the excess iron simply involves donating blood once a month. This test is the one most frequently done in our Molecular Diagnostic Lab [in Edmonton, Canada], where prenatal diagnosis accounts for only 5% of the case load…" (Wevrick 1999).

With regard to genetic testing, including that done after birth, the distinction between dominant and recessive genes is relevant (see under "hereditary diseases" in the Introduction, above). Carrying a recessive gene from only one parent regarding a hereditary disorder does not mean that one has or ever will have the disease. Of note, it is estimated that each of us carries from four to eight defective genes of some kind (Varga 1984, 84). Having an "abnormal" gene or genes or even having a genetic disease does not mean that one is an abnormal person. With regard to this, Asch and Geller raise a few pertinent questions: Will genetics continue to label people as "one of us" or "different"? Will this be intensified by the Human Genome Initiative? What is the consequence of being labeled different? (Asch and Geller 1996, 321–23).

FORENSIC GENETIC TESTING

Forensic genetic testing or "DNA fingerprinting" is now being used in many criminal investigations to identify criminals from even minute samples of blood, sperm or other bodily tissue left at the scene of a crime (Roy et al. 1994, 439). In England a genetic database has operated since 1995. More than 360,000 gene prints are now online. In the fall of 1998 the FBI activated its DNA Index System, which contains the gene prints of 250,000 convicted felons as well as 4,600 DNA samples left behind at the scenes of unsolved crimes. FBI sampling does not look at a person's entire genome but at a number of tiny stretches of DNA coding. If nine ministrands match a suspect's, the likelihood that the police have the right person is one billion to one. FBI sampling rules require no fewer than thirteen matches, which mean an even higher likelihood of having the right person. In England as many as 500 matches are made a week between database entries and samples taken from crime scenes. The FBI's new system has already helped solve 200 outstanding cases. Although some raise concerns regarding DNA fingerprinting and the rights of suspects and criminals, it should be noted that this technology has also helped innocent people. For example, in the United States DNA evidence has led to a number of convictions being overturned, including at least ten inmates on death-row being spared execution (Jeffrey Kluger in *Time* 1999, 46).

Genetic testing after birth also raises other issues. For example, it is already being used in the courts not only as a forensic tool to match crimes and criminals, but also to settle some other disputes. A couple of examples are: testing a parent in a custody case to see if he or she has Huntington's disease, which might impair his or her ability to care for his or her children; and a manufacturer demanding that an ill person be tested to determine whether or not his or her illness was caused by a toxic substance or by his or her genetic predisposition. Genetic tests after birth could also be done without the person knowing since we all regularly lose body hair and skin that contain our DNA. This is one of the themes in the movie *Gattaca*. In the future a certain type of biochip may be able to analyze a person's DNA in seconds (Golden 1999, 41–43). Some questions of consent, confidentiality and who has a right to genetic information will be treated in 2 (B) below.

(4) GENETIC TESTING BEFORE MARRIAGE AND CONCEPTION

On the island of Cyprus many people are carriers of beta-thalassemia, a single-gene recessive disease. The Greek Orthodox archbishop there has passed a ruling that couples present a certificate attesting that they have undergone carrier testing for thalassemia, as a condition for church marriage. The reason for this ruling is to give couples considering marriage more options, such as marrying another person if both tested positive as carriers, or turning to adoption rather than pregnancy, prenatal diagnosis and selective abortion (Roy et al. 1994, 172–73). The Orthodox Jewish Congregations of America support screening for Tay-Sachs disease, but only when competent guidance regarding Jewish law is provided for all participants. The Association of Orthodox Jewish Scientists endorses voluntary screening for young adults considering marriage but before definitive marriage commitments have been made (Rosner 1991, 175–76). Tay-Sachs occurs predominantly in families of Eastern European Jewish origin. It is likely that a growing number of people will want their prospective spouse screened (Rifkin 1998, 135–37).

William May thinks that persons considering marriage ought to consider the well-being of their potential children, a future generation. A person who is a carrier of a particular genetic defect possibly ought not contemplate marriage with someone who is a carrier of the same genetic defect, but rather with someone else. With regard to this he notes that the rules of many societies and the church concerning marriage between close relatives seem to be related to experience that there is a greater likelihood of children with hereditary disorders if the parents are closely related (May 1977, 118; cf., e.g., the biblical prohibitions against incest in Lev 18:5–17). Agneta Sutton, however, argues against society implementing restrictions concerning marriages between two people who together risk passing a serious genetic disease to any children they may have. She says such restrictions "would constitute a serious infringement of what is in our society a generally recognized right, namely the individual's right to marry and found a family with a partner of his or her choice" (Sutton 1995, 79; cf. USCC 1996).

Concerning responsible parenthood Pope Paul VI in *Humanae Vitae* teaches in part:

> In relation to physical, economic, psychological and social conditions, responsible parenthood is exercised, either by the deliberate and generous decision to raise a numerous family, or by the decision, made for grave motives and with due respect for the moral law, to avoid for the time being, or even for an indeterminate period, a new birth.
>
> The responsible exercise of parenthood implies, therefore, that husband and wife recognize fully their own duties towards God, towards themselves, towards the family and towards society, in a correct hierarchy of values. (Paul VI 1968, n. 10)

Although this Catholic teaching does not specifically address questions of couples who face the possibility of having children with serious genetic disorders, it is relevant to such questions.

Benedict Ashley and Kevin O'Rourke point out that there are some risks of defect for *every* child. Thus all prospective parents are faced with the issue of whether or not they have the capacity to care for a potentially defective child with the reasonable help of society. As in other areas of life, people should accept and meet reasonable risks. Married couples should not have the attitude that they will only have children if they are perfect and require the least care possible. None of us is perfect. Giving life to a new human being is a great thing, a blessing (cf. Gen 1:28). On the basis of objective information, including information about the social resources that may be available to them, individuals and couples should make their own decisions about having children. "...[I]f the risks are high, such as 25 percent, of begetting a child so defective as to require care that the parents cannot supply, even with reasonable and available social assistance, then they have the responsibility to consider not begetting children." Such a difficult decision should not imply that any human life is not worth living. If married couples have serious reasons to try to avoid conceiving a child, Ashley and O'Rourke agree with Catholic teaching that methods of contraception and sterilization are immoral, whereas periodic abstinence or natural family planning (NFP) can be moral. Newer methods of NFP, including the Ovulation Method and the Sympto-Thermal Method, have proven to be highly effective. In any case, if a child is already conceived, no reason justifies directly destroying it (Ashley and O'Rourke 1997, 329–30 and Ch. 10).

Regarding Catholic teaching on birth control see Paul VI (1968) and John Paul II (1981, nn. 28–35). Among other things, Pope John Paul II speaks of anti-life mentalities resulting from "the absence in people's hearts of God, whose love alone is stronger than all the world's fears and can conquer them" and "the Church firmly believes that human life, even if weak and suffering, is always a splendid gift of God's goodness" (John Paul II 1981, n. 30).

Concerning questions of the mentally disabled getting married and having children see Jean Vanier (1985, Chs. 5–8).

Andrew Varga thinks society should not set standards of normalcy regarding responsible parenthood and the possibility of having children with defects. "Genetic defects in themselves do not make a person abnormal." One should not only consider the possible difficulties and sufferings of a child, but also the joys and the value of his or her life. Nobody can conclude that any life is "not worth living." Nevertheless, if the probability is very high of a couple having very defective offspring and they are not capable of taking care of such children with the appropriate help of society, he thinks they should abstain from having children (Varga 1984, 87–88). Married couples who have non-selfish reasons for not procreating their own biological children, like those who are unable to procreate children, could consider the possibility of adopting children.

With regard to these issues the following policy of the Medical Research Council of Canada is relevant: "The freedom of couples who are at risk to plan and carry potentially affected pregnancies [i.e., with a genetic disorder], and the support of children and adults with handicapping conditions, should not be compromised" (MRCC et al. 1998, 8.5).

The Vatican's Pontifical Academy for Life has said (October 1999) that, "Post-natal genetic diagnosis—disease-screening for people getting married, applying for a job, or deciding to have children, for example—is morally licit under certain conditions. It must benefit the physical and emotional health of the individual undergoing the test; it must not be used as a discriminatory method; the subject must give his or her consent; the individual's privacy must be respected; and the diagnosis of genetic disease must be presented to the subject only when he or she has reached adulthood" (Thavis 1999, 5).

2.B. Genetic Counseling, Confidentiality and Discrimination

Among other things, confusion and uncertainties regarding genetic tests, including how genetic disorders express themselves and what role environment plays, can lead many people to make uninformed decisions. This includes thousands of parents making decisions concerning their unborn children (Rifkin 1998, 134). This underscores the need for accurate information and good genetic counseling. The Code of Ethics of the National Society of Genetic Counselors states that genetic counselors should strive to "enable their clients to make informed independent decisions, free of coercion, by providing or illuminating the necessary facts and clarifying the alternatives and anticipated consequences" (NSGC 1992, II.3). Ideally, good genetic counseling should be provided both before genetic testing, to help people considering a genetic test to determine whether or not possible benefits outweigh possible risks, and after genetic testing, to help those involved to understand properly the results and their options (Ashley and O'Rourke 1997, 327–29).

Counselors and geneticists themselves are divided over several issues, for example: how should they respond to a request for prenatal diagnosis only to determine the sex of the child (i.e., regarding possible sex-selective abortion); whether or not they should always tell the whole truth (e.g., if communicating certain information would not seem to provide any benefits and may psychologically disturb the person seeking counseling, such as a woman unable to conceive due to a sex chromosome anomaly that cannot be fixed); and whether or not it is ever justifiable to disclose information to third parties. With regard to the latter the Canadian College of Medical Geneticists (CCMG) directs counselors "to keep information obtained from patients in confidence, unless patients have given written permission to release this information to others, or unless it can be shown that nondisclosure of this information is likely to cause significant harm to the health of other persons" (Roy et al. 1994, 175. Cf. NSGC 1992, II.5; CMA 1996, nn. 22–24; USCC 1994, n. 34; and CHAC 2000, 33 and 65). With regard to Huntington's disease, when a person diagnosed as having the disease refuses to tell siblings who have a fifty percent chance of carrying the gene, some Canadian geneticists would respect confidentiality whereas others would utilize the CCMG exception clause cited above (Roy et al. 1994, 176).

The Principle of Professional Communications, as formulated by Ashley and O'Rourke, is relevant to these issues:

To fulfill their obligations to serve patients, health care professionals have the responsibility to:

1. Strive to establish and preserve trust at both the emotional and rational levels.
2. Share the information they possess that is legitimately needed by others in order to have an informed conscience.
3. Refrain from lying or giving misinformation.
4. Keep information secret that is not legitimately needed by others and that if revealed might harm the patient, others, or destroy trust. (Ashley and O'Rourke 1994, 41–42)

With regard to n. 2, health care professionals, including genetic counselors, should first of all provide their patients/clients with the information they need for informed consent, that is, "all information that would be useful to a reasonable person in the same circumstance..." (CHAC 1991, 31. Cf. CMA 1996, nn. 12–21). They should also provide their patients/clients as well as others the information they each legitimately need to have an informed conscience to carry out their respective responsibilities. On the other hand, all persons capable of such have a responsibility "to inform themselves as fully as possible about the facts and ethical norms of a particular issue and to act according to this well-informed conscience. ...Catholics, in addition, are morally bound to inform themselves of the teachings of the Church regarding moral issues" (CHAC 1991, 14; cf. USCC 1994, nn. 23–28; and CHAUSA 1990. For a fuller explanation of principles related to developing a well-formed conscience, see, e.g., Ashley and O'Rourke 1997, 182–86). With regard to relevant facts, including one's alternatives and norms or principles, one should also try to discern what values are relevant and what proper appreciation and respect of these values requires (see Chs. 3 and 4 below).

Today, due to our family history, we may realize that we have a significant chance of carrying a serious genetic defect that we may pass on to our children, or of having a genetic disease such as Huntington's disease, which later in life would lead to progressive deterioration and premature death. Ashley and O'Rourke think that individuals who have good reason to "suspect they have such serious defects would be wise to have the matter settled by a reliable test [provided such is available] and to adjust their life plans accordingly." Nevertheless, individuals in such situations "should have the freedom to decide whether they wish a diagnosis" (Ashley and O'Rourke 1997, 330).

Without proper protection of confidentiality, David J. Roy, John R. Williams and Bernard M. Dickens think that there is a danger that an increase in presymptomatic genetic testing could lead to an increase in stigmatization, ostracization and unfair discrimination. For example, people might be denied, on the basis of their genotype, access to education, insurance, employment and other opportunities and services that are supposed to be open to all in society (Roy et al. 1994, 452–55; cf. the movie *Gattica*).

There have already been some cases of genetic discrimination by insurance companies and employers. In one case, a family's coverage was canceled when the insurance company discovered that one of its four children was afflicted with fragile X disease. In the light of such cases and related concerns, laws have been passed in some places to "exclude insurers from discriminating on the basis of genetic predispositions." Such legislation, however, has been opposed by the insurance industry with arguments such as that the industry "needs to be able to use genetic information, like all other medical information, in deciding whether or not to insure some-one and at what price" (Rifkin 1998, 161–62). The U.S. Health Insurance Portability and Accountability Act of 1996 is an example of legislation that "prohibits group health plans from denying indi-viduals coverage on the basis of genetic information, or using such information to charge them higher rates…." Insurance companies, however, "fear that genetically compromised persons will purchase added insurance" (Kaveny 1999, 143; for more information on U.S. policy and legislation see ELSI).

With regard to employee discrimination, in one case an employer abruptly dismissed a social worker on learning that she was at risk of developing Huntington's disease since some of her family members had developed the illness. She herself was not symptomatic nor had she ever been tested for the disease. In the light of such concerns Rifkin argues that "laws will have to be established in every country to prohibit employers from discriminating against human beings whom they regard as 'genetically less fit' for certain tasks based on predispositions that may or may not manifest themselves, and even if they do, may not seriously compromise an individual's ability to 'get the job done'" (Rifkin 1998, 164–65). The Americans with Disabili-ties Act of 1990 has been understood "to prohibit employers from taking into account genetic information about asymptomatic applicants when making job offers…" (Kaveny 1999, 143; for more information on U.S. policy and legislation, see ELSI).

With regard to genetic discrimination, we can note here that the Medical Research Council of Canada says that the results of genetic testing and genetic counseling records should be protected from access by third parties, unless free and informed consent is given by the subject, and the subject should be informed of any limits of confidentiality. Misunderstanding or misuse of the results of genetic tests can affect not only an individual's opportunities, but also his or her identity and self-worth and stigmatize the entire group to which the individual belongs (MRCC et al. 1998, 8.1–2; cf. John Paul II 1995a, 82).

There has been a lot of legal and ethical discussion regarding whether or not genetic counseling should be or can be non-directive. The Medical Research Council of Canada says genetic counselors have two main roles in dealing with a family: "The first is to educate regarding the condition in question, and the second is to counsel by presenting options or possible action scenarios in a non-directive manner. The complexity of genetic information and its social implications usually requires that free and informed consent be supplemented with genetic counselling." In genetic research "counseling regarding the potential benefits, harms and limitations of each study is crucial both before the individual gives free and informed consent and after results are available." Researchers and counselors should also understand important cultural issues regarding genetic inheritance and discrimination (MRCC et al. 1998, 8.4).

According to Roy, Williams and Dickens, most genetic counselors in Canada see their role primarily as information-givers regarding various options, as support-givers, and not to provide ethical analysis, but to be non-directive and non-judgmental (Roy et al. 1994, 174). Andrew Varga, however, says that most people who undergo genetic tests want not only an interpretation of the data but also moral guidance in their decision. The ethical part of genetic counseling is not an easy task. Unfortunately, "it surpasses the training and educational background of most genetic counselors." He hopes that more counselors would be educated "who can understand the concrete ethical problems of the counselees. Counselors should be morally sensitive and intellectually capable of giving prudent advice so that the counselees can make their own ethically responsible decisions" (Varga 1984, 88–89). Good ethical counseling helps people to form their consciences properly, taking into account not only the relevant options and facts, but also the relevant values and norms (ethical, legal and professional). It helps people to make truly informed decisions that they are less likely to regret later. Providing good ethical counseling does not mean being judgmental of people (cf. Matt 7:1–5, and John 8:1–11).

Counselors' perceptions of their own objectivity is not a good indication of what actually happens, according to Dr. Dorothy Wertz, senior scientist for the Shriver Center for Mental Retardation. People with disabilities generally rate their own quality of life much higher than their caregivers. Genetic counselors may share the caregivers' perceptions or be even less informed. She says the trend worldwide is for counselors to provide purposely slanted information, much of it pessimistic, or to give directive advice. This is less prevalent in English-speaking countries, but she predicts they will soon catch up as physicians take over more counseling from geneticists. "A lot of them make no bones about suggesting abortion...you have no comeback. They're the experts." She also says that the most pessimistic brochures on diseases come from commercial companies. "If you're trying to market tests, you don't want to say you can have a rich, rewarding life if you have cystic fibrosis." Instead you paint a bleak picture (Elliott 1998, 6). Medical anthropologist Nancy Press thinks it is morally wrong that many pamphlets (the only source of genetic information for most women) that are routinely handed out in the course of prenatal care sugarcoat the message with language such as "having a better birth outcome" instead of being clear that the test is really about selective termination, that is, abortion (Golden 1999, 43). In a documentary, a number of disabled people interviewed share how others often rate their quality of life poorly whereas they are quite happy. One of those interviewed, Connie Panzarino, has a genetic neurological disease as well as a Master's degree. She says that women, couples and families receiving genetic counseling are not getting informed choice since disabled people are not being asked to counsel them. Disabled people are the only ones who have that information (CBC 1992).

With regard to the frequent link between genetic testing, counseling and abortion, it should be noted that others besides the woman who requests an abortion and the doctor who performs it may have committed gravely illicit acts. Concerning this the Vatican's Congregation for the Doctrine of the Faith says:

> The spouse or relatives or anyone else would similarly be acting in a manner contrary to the moral law if they were to counsel or impose such a diagnostic procedure on the expectant mother with the same intention of possibly proceeding to an abortion. So too the specialist would be guilty of illicit collaboration if, in conducting the diagnosis and in communicating its results, he were deliberately to contribute to establishing or favoring a link between prenatal diagnosis and abortion....any directive or program of the civil and health authorities or of scientific organizations which in any way were to favor a link between prenatal diagnosis and abortion...is to be condemned as a violation of the unborn child's right to life... (CDF 1987, I.2).

Ashley and O'Rourke argue not only that counselors should not recommend abortion as a solution, but that even if the parents declare an intention to abort, the counselor should not cooperate with them. Counselors should try to protect the rights of the fetus to life, as they would protect the rights of a child already born, against infringement of these rights by the parents:

> A counselor, however, in doing whatever possible to avoid abortion, should exercise great prudence, avoiding threats, pressures, and recriminations, since these will only aggravate the situation. Indeed, undue persuasion may lead to a malpractice claim....In sum, if abortion is in question, the counselor should respect the conscience of the parents while doing everything possible to protect the child.

They think that counselors should provide parents with information to which they have a right, even if they suspect the parents may use the information for purposes such as abortion that the counselor considers unethical. They also think that Catholic health care facilities have a duty to provide genetic counseling "in accordance with Christian moral standards, since otherwise parents will be forced to obtain information from centers where abortion will be an accepted and even encouraged solution" (Ashley and O'Rourke 1997, 328–29; cf. USCC 1994, n. 54; and CHAUSA 1990. For some principles with regard to cooperation see also Ashley and O'Rourke 1997, 193–99; CHAC 2000, 13–14 and Appendix II; and USCC 1994, nn. 45–46 and the Appendix). With regard to the views expressed above that one should not intend or promote the wrongdoing of another, we can note that Jesus taught that not only outwardly harmful acts such as murder and adultery are wrong. One can also sin in one's heart by merely intending such (see Matt 5:21–28). It seems to me that the Golden Rule, Jesus' teaching to "always treat others as you would like them to treat you," is also relevant to the various questions concerning genetic counseling that have been raised here.

2. C. Genetic Therapy

Genetic therapy involves the use of recombinant DNA technology (see the Introduction) to treat diseases involving missing or defective genes. Genetic therapy could involve inserting a normal gene or DNA sequence into targeted cells to produce a needed protein that would normally be produced by the missing or defective gene or DNA sequence. In the future it could also involve genetic "surgery," removing a defective gene or DNA segment and replacing it with its normal equivalent. With regard to genetic therapy, many today speak of two main types. Somatic gene therapy would only affect body cells, not reproductive cells. It would only affect the individual treated, not his or her offspring. Germ-line gene therapy, however, would affect reproductive cells in the individual and thus affect any offspring he or she may have (O'Calllaghan, 25–26; Suzuki and Knudtson 1988, Ch. 8). Advances in genetics could also be used in other therapeutic ways such as to design new drugs, vaccines and sources of replacement tissues for human beings.

SOMATIC GENE THERAPY

Somatic gene therapy is widely approved in theory for proportionate reasons, especially if there is no other effective treatment. With regard to this, one would consider the expected or hoped-for benefits of the genetic therapy for the individual, as compared to the expected or feared risks. One would also compare the expected benefits and harms of any other treatment options and of no treatment at all.

The first human somatic gene therapy was carried out in 1990 by Dr. French Anderson and his team on two girls with ADA deficiency (see the Introduction). Although this experiment was hailed a success by the media, some scientists have questioned its degree of effectiveness. Since then experiments have been carried out on hundreds of people with various diseases such as cystic fibrosis, hemophilia and muscular dystrophy. Although some experiments have produced varying degrees of success, "to date, no one has found a way to reliably control the therapeutic genes to make them clinically useful." With regard to risks, it should be noted that a genetic therapy trial at the University of Pennsylvania unexpectedly led to the death of an eighteen-year-old Arizona man, Jesse Gelsinger, with a rare genetic liver disease, ornithine transcarbamylase deficiency, on September 16, 1999. Following this, the United States Food and Drug Administration shut down eight gene therapy trials at that university. In February 2000 legislation was introduced into the United States House of Representatives to tighten up the regulation of federally-funded human gene therapy trials (The Associated Press, 1999; and BioNews Jan. 31, and Feb. 14, 2000). Nevertheless, many scientists in the field are convinced that somatic gene therapies will bear more fruit as knowledge and procedures improve (Kmiec 1999; cf. Rifkin 1998, 129–31; and Wilson 1999). Since somatic gene therapy is a relatively young science, proper caution should be taken in long-term monitoring of results, and in counseling and consent procedures. In the light of limited successes to date, it is important to avoid creating unrealistic expectations (SRT 1998, "Moral and Ethical Issues in Gene Therapy").

Canada's Royal Commission on New Reproductive Technologies concluded that somatic cell gene therapy may be appropriate in some situations (RCNRT 1993, 17). The Medical Research Council of Canada says that somatic gene therapy may be considered for approval. Since we lack information regarding possible long-term harms gene alteration should only be undertaken in "the context of well-defined serious single gene conditions or malignancies." Gene alteration is irreversible. "The potential risks of gene alteration include reinfectivity and oncogenicity of the viral vector, interruption of a normal host gene with negative consequences, bacterial contamination, establishment of the inserted gene in germ cells with unanticipated consequences, and only partial correction of the genetic disease, thus converting a fatal condition to a chronic progressive one" (MRCC et al. 1998, 8.5; cf. AMA 1996, "E-2.11 Gene Therapy").

With regard to somatic gene therapy, the following statement by Pope John Paul II is relevant:

> A strictly therapeutic intervention whose explicit objective is the healing of various maladies such as those stemming from deficiencies of chromosomes will, in principle, be considered desirable, provided it is directed to the true promotion of the personal well-being of man and does not infringe on his integrity or worsen his conditions of life. Such an intervention, indeed, would fall within the logic of the Christian moral tradition." (John Paul II 1983; cf. CHAUSA 1990)

A number of other Christians who address the issue of somatic gene therapy generally concur that it can be ethical for proportionate reasons. James Walters notes that, "Nearly all the task forces, ecclesial communities, and individual theologians who have addressed... somatic cell therapy, have approved of its use once the scientific and technical difficulties have been solved" (Walter 2000, 125; cf., e.g., Thavis 1999, 5; Sutton 1995, 83–84; Hoose 1995, 56; Rodriguez 2000, 36; and SRT 1998, "Moral and Ethical Issues in Gene Therapy"). Thomas Shannon thinks that somatic gene therapy should also be considered and debated in the context of resource allocation and priorities, since it will cost a lot to develop such therapies and other health needs are increasing (Shannon 2000, 116–17).

GERM-LINE GENE THERAPY

Germ-line gene therapy is widely disapproved of or at least seen as too risky to attempt on human beings given the present limits of human knowledge in this area. In 1983 religious leaders and prominent scientists in the United States urged a worldwide ban on human germ-line therapy experiments (Rifkin 1998, 131). Because of serious medical risks, not only to the individual treated but also to his or her offspring and future generations, "there is at present a world-wide moratorium on this kind of therapy" (Sutton 1995, 84). Nevertheless, since further research, including germ-line research on animals and research on artificial chromosomes, may reduce some of these risks in the future (Reuters 1999), it is worthwhile to consider some of the arguments that have been raised both for and against this therapy.

Arguments raised in support of human germ-line research and therapy include the following: if successful, germ-line gene therapy would reduce or eliminate the risks of people, that either have certain diseases such as Huntington's disease or are carriers of genes for certain diseases such as thalassemia, transmitting these to their children, such people and their offspring could procreate with less concern. If perhaps germ-line gene therapy could eventually eliminate certain diseases from certain families, or even from the human gene pool, this would prevent much human suffering. It could also significantly reduce health care costs in the long run, including the costs of somatic gene therapy in successive generations. R. Munson and L. H. Davis argue that the conceivability of disasters "does not warrant refusing to develop these techniques for eliminating genetic diseases." They suggest that perhaps some day the survival of the human race will depend on germ-line genetic manipulations (Munson and Davis 1992, 151–52). Some also argue that individuals should have the freedom of choice to have their body parts altered including their reproductive cells. In the light of such arguments, even though the consequences of attempting human germ-line therapy are very unpredictable, Rifkin says a growing number of molecular biologists, medical practitioners and pharmaceutical companies are willing to take the gamble (Rifkin 1998, 132–33; cf. Sutton 1995, 84–85; and Shannon 2000, 117).

Arguments raised against human germ-line research and therapy include the following: first of all, "the risks involved concern not only the individual treated but also his offspring." "…the price to be paid for any mishaps would be high, since these would be hereditary and transmitted from one generation to the next. Furthermore, germ-line therapy means treating or subjecting future generations to today's techniques, techniques that may seem crude and simple by tomorrow's standards." Even if germ-line therapy was capable of ridding certain families or humankind of certain diseases, "there would always be new mutations, and some of the old diseases would turn up *de novo* in new generations" (Sutton 1995, 84).

Canada's Royal Commission on New Reproductive Technologies concluded that research on germ-line genetic alteration should not be conducted in Canada since this is not the only way to avoid having affected offspring, and "there are many potential harms, without clear benefit to any individual" (RCNRT 1993, 17). The Medical Research Council of Canada also concludes that gene alteration involving human germ-line cells or human embryos "is not ethically acceptable" (MRCC et al. 1998, 8.5). Germ-line and early embryo gene therapy is at present legally prohibited in the United Kingdom. Dr. Donald Bruce argues that this is appropriate with our current state of genetic knowledge. Even if human germ-line therapy ever became technically feasible, "the technical difficulties, risks and cost involved in applying it on the scale which would be needed to eliminate a given gene from a population would be simply prohibitive" (SRT 1998, "Moral and Ethical Issues in Gene Therapy"; cf. Shannon 2000, 117–18).

Some argue that eliminating genetic disorders at the germ-line would result in a dangerous narrowing of the human gene pool upon which future generations rely for making evolutionary adaptations to changing environments. Rifkin notes that many molecular biologists speak of mutations and genetic diseases as "errors" in the code (compare bugs in a computer program), whereas evolutionary biologists view them as variations in a theme—a rich reservoir of genetic diversity essential to maintaining the viability of a species. Eliminating certain disease genes could also result in the loss of certain good traits. For example, the sickle-cell recessive trait protects against malaria and the cystic fibrosis recessive gene may play a role in protecting against cholera. We are just beginning to learn the many subtle and varied roles recessive genes play. "To think of recessive traits and single gene disorders, then, as merely errors in the code, in need of reprogramming, is to lose sight of how things really work in the biological kingdom" (Rifkin 1998, 144–46; cf. Sutton 1995, 84).

Making changes at the germ-line would involve engineering the human species much like engineering a piece of machinery. Engineers seek to perfect machines. When one set of defects is eliminated they turn their attention to the next set of defects. Commonly used language regarding genetics such as "defect" and "abnormality" presupposes an image of perfection. Germ-line gene therapy would set humanity on a course of seeking to create "an unattainable new archetype, a flawless, errorless, perfect being to which to aspire." Since every human being carries a number of lethal recessive genes all of us could be seen as "riddled with errors in our code." Many disabled people are becoming increasingly frightened that people like themselves will be seen as defective, mistakes, errors in the code to be eliminated (Rifkin 1998 145–47; cf. CBC 1992).

Some also argue that germ-line gene therapy would violate a person's right to natural DNA, a genome that has not been tampered with, an unchanged genetic inheritance. Modifying the genetic structure of "as-yet-unconceived individuals" would amount to "playing God" (O'Callaghan 1994, 26–27). Taking into account human folly, Paul Ramsey does not think that "man is or will ever be wise enough to make himself a successful self-modifying system or wise enough to begin doctoring the species" (Ramsey 1970, 123–24). Germ-line therapy would mean "exercising a new form of control over future generations" without their consent. It would foster a producer and consumer attitude toward children, asking for babies with or without certain qualities. With this there is the social and moral risk "that the value of children will be measured in units of health and performance quality, social utility and parental satisfaction. That is to say, there is the risk that their intrinsic value and dignity as human beings, as our neighbors and fellow images of God will tend to be forgotten" (Sutton 1995, 85). In an address to members of the World Medical Association, Pope John Paul II does not speak of germ-line therapy by name, but he does speak of respecting the fundamental dignity of people and "avoiding manipulations that tend to modify genetic inheritance" (1983). The Vatican's Pontifical Academy for Life has said (October 1999) that "germ-line gene therapy...is ethically unacceptable because it involves a high-risk technique used on embryos, usually coupled with *in vitro* fertilization. It also poses a long-term risk to future generations" (Thavis 1999, 5; cf. Rodriguez 2000, 31 and 36).

Along with advances in genetics, the pharmaceutical industry is exploding with ideas to design new drugs. Much research is already being done and is expected to be done in the coming decades to design new drugs with the help of gene-based science and technologies. While genetic therapy would target disorders at the genetic level, genetically engineered drugs would have other targets such as RNA molecules which transfer information from genes to proteins, or the proteins and enzymes themselves. In the future drugs are expected to be safer, more powerful and much more selective than ever before. It is also expected that someday doctors will be able to consult a person's genetic profile to determine ahead of time how a person is likely to respond to various medications. This whole area holds much promise for developing more effective treatments with less side effects for various cancers, Alzheimer's, AIDS and other diseases (Christine Gorman in *Time* 1999, 57–61). Developments in genetics are also expected to lead to developing more effective vaccines and producing certain vaccines in genetically engineered plants that could be eaten. Genetic developments may also lead to other therapeutic developments such as producing healthy replacement tissue from stem cells (see 2.E.2 below), or even staving off the aging process (Michael Lemonick, Alice Park and Clare Thompson in *Time* 1999, 69–70).

2.D. Genetic Design and Enhancement

Genetic design and enhancement engineering, unlike genetic therapy, would not be intended to prevent or cure diseases. Genetic design would mean deliberately designing a human being by choosing the genetic material he or she would have in the attempt to modify or produce certain desired traits. This could involve choosing for certain traits such as sex, tallness, skin color, music ability, and so forth. Genetic enhancement would involve seeking to improve people genetically, for example, "by making them better looking, more artistic or more intelligent or athletic" (Sutton 1995, 85). Ultimately, we might be able to produce human beings by recipe, even with DNA combinations that have never existed before, although this is futuristic and may only be a remote possibility. Nevertheless, what is already being done with regard to the genetic engineering of plants and animals (see Ch. 1 above) can give us some idea of the possibilities for genetically engineering human beings.

SEX SELECTION

Sex selection is one of the simplest forms of such engineering. In Chapter 2.A above we have already considered sex selection by means of prenatal diagnosis and selective abortion, and preimplantation diagnosis and zygote or embryo selection. There also exist certain preconception techniques of sex selection that do not involve the moral issues of abortion and discarding unwanted embryos, but that still involve certain moral issues. These involve certain techniques to increase the chances of either a Y sex chromosome carrying sperm to fertilize an ovum to produce a boy, or an X sex chromosome carrying sperm to fertilize an ovum to produce a girl. The microsort method attempts to separate sperm by size using flow cytometry. Y carrying sperm are a bit smaller and lighter than X carrying sperm. Another technique developed by Dr. Ronald Ericsson attempts to separate sperm by having them swim through albumen. Y carrying sperm generally swim faster than X carrying sperm. A third method advocated by Landrum Shettles, M.D., uses timing of intercourse: a couple wanting to increase their chances of having a boy would wait until the time of ovulation (determined by means such as the Billings Method of Natural Family Planning) to have intercourse, since Y carrying sperm generally swim faster; a couple wanting to increase their chances of having a girl would have intercourse up until three days before ovulation, since Y carrying sperm generally live longer. Supporters of these methods claim success rates of up to 80 percent or so (Jick 1999, and Breckenridge 1987).

In the first two methods described above, semen would normally be obtained by the man masturbating and by transferring the preferred group of sperm into the woman's reproductive tract by artificial insemination. Many Christian ethicists approve of artificial insemination within a healthy marriage for proportionate reasons. Catholic teaching and ethicists who agree with this teaching, however, consider masturbation and artificial insemination which substitutes for the conjugal act to be immoral because they voluntarily dissociate the two meanings of the conjugal act: the reciprocal total self-giving unitive meaning and the procreative meaning. On the other hand, Catholic teaching holds that "if the technical means facilitates the conjugal act or helps it to reach its natural objectives, it can be morally acceptable" (CDF 1987, II.6. For a fuller discussion of artificial means of assisting human procreation see, e.g., CDF 1987, II; USCC 1994, Part 4; CHAC 2000, 40–41; Ashley and O'Rourke 1997, Ch. 9.2; and May 2000, Ch. 3.). The third method of preconception sex selection described above, timing intercourse for this purpose, would avoid the ethical problems of masturbation and artificial insemination, but it would still involve ethical issues related to sex selection per se.

Couples could use sex selection techniques for various motives. For example, one or both of them prefers to have a boy or a girl or to have a certain birth order. A couple who already has boys or girls may want to foster gender balance within their family. Having a boy in some places (e.g., China and India) may have economic or other advantages. And, if only the mother is carrying an X-linked genetic disorder such as hemophilia or Duchenne's muscular dystrophy, fifty percent of her male children will have the disease, whereas none of her female children will have the disease. Fifty percent of her female children, however, would be carriers of the disorder.

Nature provides an approximately fifty/fifty human sex ratio at the age of marriage. This gender balance has been upset to some extent by the use of sex selection techniques in some places, including China and India. This has negative consequences with regard to appreciating the value of women, and the value of male/female companionship and marriage. This might not happen in countries such as the United States and Canada where the great majority of people do not have a bias with respect to the sex of their children. Nevertheless, Canada's Royal Commission on New Reproductive Technologies concluded that "sex-selective insemination services should not be available in Canada for reasons of sex preference." It recommended that "such services be provided only where there is a medical indication such as an X-linked disorder..." (RCNRT 1993, 16; cf. Hoose 1995, 59–60). With regard to the morality of seeking to avoid conceiving a child with a serious genetic disorder see the related discussion in 2.A.4 above.

Canada's Royal Commission considered sex selection, simply because one sex is preferred over the other, whatever the means, to be "incompatible with Canadian values." Among other things, such sex selection "reinforces the idea that the sex of a child is important, and encourages the view that families with all boys or all girls are less than ideal"; "it could make existing children in the family feel that their own sex was lacking in some way"; and "it would involve an inappropriate use of resources" (RCNRT 1993, 16). Varga says that sex selection "carries with it the danger of the children becoming simply means for certain goals of the parents." Additional tension might also be caused in the family "when the spouses cannot agree upon the sex of their children" (Varga 1984, 248–49). With regard to sex selection, Ashley and O'Rourke say that "it is important to children to be accepted by their parents as a divine gift to be loved for what they uniquely are and not merely because they conform to the parents' hopes or expectations." This consideration also "applies to more complex forms of genetic reconstruction" (Ashley and O'Rourke 1994, 184).

OTHER KINDS OF GENETIC DESIGN AND ENHANCEMENT

Other kinds of genetic design and enhancement could conceivably be done with recombinant DNA technology. These could involve somatic cell modifications that would not be passed on or germ-line modifications that would be passed on to future generations. Used for purposes of genetic design or enhancement these would raise some of the same issues as genetic therapy (see 2.C above). Genetic design and enhancement, however, also raise additional questions such as: what are "desirable" or "superior" human traits? Since it would be naive to expect all people to agree on this, who should decide? Jeremy Rifkin thinks that one of the most troubling political questions in all of human history is: to whom should we entrust authority to decide what is a good gene and what is a bad gene? Should we entrust this authority to scientists, corporations, governments, other institutions, parents, other groups of individuals and/or consumers? (Rifkin 1998, 172).

Since a person's personality depends on all his or her "intellectual, emotive, affective and other mental and spiritual characteristics working together," Agneta Sutton asks, "Who are we to alter this inter-play? What could possibly make anyone think that it is for us to decide that it would be better for a child to be given a certain gene conferring on it, say, greater mathematical or musical ability?" She points out that the hoped-for genius "may turn out to be devoid of all feeling or to be a Frankenstein monster" (Sutton 1995, 86). Concerning this we can also consider the story (no doubt apocryphal) of the dancer Isadora Duncan and the writer Bernard Shaw. She suggested that they "make babies" since the children would have her beautiful body and his magnificent mind. Shaw, however, responded, "Yes, but what if they had *my* body and *your* brains?" (May 1977, 71; Rollinson 1999, C.3).

Shannon observes that the genetic enhancement debate is "characterized by an unacknowledged genetic determinism," which assumes that "all behaviors, no matter how complex," are caused by genes. This neglects the role of environment in developing our characteristics (Shannon 2000, 118–19). It also neglects the role of human free will and God's grace.

Some who argue in favor of genetic design and enhancement say there is no discernible line between genetic therapy and improvement. As discussed above (2.C), many favor genetic therapy, at least somatic gene therapy for proportionate reasons, to treat diseases that cause serious mental impairments, physical disabilities and/or premature death. If clinicians and parents are allowed to do this for children to prevent or cure major defects, some ask, why not also for less serious medical problems and learning disabilities? And if for these, why say no to modifications that would increase a healthy child's intelligence, memory, verbal skills, athletic ability, height, life span, and so on? (Michael Lemonick and Robert Wright in *Time* 1999, 48–51; Barnard 1999). With regard to this issue, consider the case of a new genetically engineered growth hormone. This was originally marketed in the 1980s in the United States for the small number of children with dwarfism. Within a few years, however, many parents were requesting and many doctors were prescribing this engineered product for shorter children who were not suffering from a growth hormone deficit. Many young men were also obtaining it illegally on the black market to enhance their muscles. Some have even begun to consider normal shortness a disease (Rifkin 1998, 139–44). With regard to this issue it is worth drawing attention, for example, to two movies, *Simon Birch* and *Rudy,* which foster an appreciation of remarkable qualities in a dwarf and a short football player, respectively.

Sutton responds to the argument that there is no clear line between cure and enhancement as follows:

> There is no clear line between talking or shouting either, yet there are definite cases of both. And most of us can see that there are such things as real illnesses, and that curing an individual child of an illness such as cystic fibrosis is very different from making sure it has the body and strength of an Olympic athlete, the mathematical and scientific intelligence of an Einstein and the voice of a Pavarotti or Maria Callas. (Sutton 1995, 86–87)

Some, for example Robert Sinsheimer and Lee Silver, envision using genetic design and enhancement in the future to direct evolution, including that of the human species (Rifkin 1998, 144 and 168–69). Catholic ethicists, Ashley and O'Rourke, say they would not rule this out "ethically merely on the grounds that it would be usurpation of God's creative power, since God wishes to share this creative power with human persons if we use it well...." With regard to this they also say in part that

> it is possible to imagine that someday in other environments it might become necessary, for example, to replace the human lungs with other ways of obtaining oxygen. In principle it would seem that such changes would be ethical (1) if they gave support to human intelligence by helping the life of the brain and (2) if they did not suppress any of the fundamental human functions that integrate the human personality.

They say that "grave ethical difficulties, however, do arise over whether society has either the knowledge or the virtue to take the responsibility for creating...[by genetic reconstruction] superior members of the race." With regard to this they conclude in part:

1. It is more feasible, technically and ethically, to improve the human condition by improving the environment and development of the individual....Priority in research and investment of medical resources should be given to [these]....

2. Presently proposed methods of genetic reconstruction of human beings involve in vitro fertilization and other procedures that are ethically objectionable because they separate reproduction from its parental context and involve the production of human beings, some of whom will be defective because of experimental failure and who probably will be destroyed....

3. Proposals to improve the human race by sex selection, cloning, or genetic reconstruction are ethically unacceptable in the present state of knowledge. Unless limited to very modest interventions, they would restrict the genetic variability important to human survival.... (Ashley and O'Rourke 1997, 318 and 322–23)

If genetic technologies became available to engineer "superior" human beings, who would take advantage of these? Since these technologies are likely to be very expensive, only wealthy people could provide these for their children and themselves. Rich people generally already provide their children with many advantages, and it is likely that some of them would also want to provide their children with genetic advantages. It also seems unlikely that our already overly burdened publically funded health care systems would provide such services, which are not therapeutic but "cosmetic," for everyone who wants them. In the light of this, molecular biologist Silver, for example, envisages a world in the not-too-distant future made up of Gen Rich and Natural classes. Others such as Rifkin, however, are concerned that attempts to engineer our own perfection may end up compromising our humanity (Rifkin 1998, 168–74; cf. Michael Lemonick and Robert Wright in *Time* 1999, 48–51). The movie *Gattaca* interestingly explores some issues related to this. Varga says that genetically engineering super human beings would

> ...create a special elite class unless the whole population is changed. Either case would mean an unethical manipulation....The manipulators would be trying to use an elite or a specially designed group of human beings as a means for their own goals. This would be a violation of the inherent right of persons for self-determination. If the "upgrading"...were to affect everybody, it is obvious that the whole population could not be changed without a massive totalitarian manipulation of every individual. This would involve the total suppression of freedom. (Varga 1984, 145)

Canada's Royal Commission on New Reproductive Technologies concluded that "genetic enhancement carries social and medical risks disproportionate to any benefit, and involves opportunity costs by diverting scarce financial and profession resources away from real medical problems. No research into this area should be permitted or funded in Canada" (RCNRT 1993, 17). The Medical Research Council of Canada says, "The aim of genetic research should be to advance knowledge or to alleviate disease, not to 'improve' or 'enhance' a population by cosmetic manipulation" (MRCC et al. 1998, 8.5).

With regard to genetic interventions that are "not strictly therapeutic," for example, "those aimed at the amelioration of the human biological condition," Pope John Paul II says in part:

> In particular, this kind of intervention must not infringe on the origin of human life, that is, procreation linked to the union, not only biological but also spiritual, of the parents, united by the bond of marriage. It must, consequently, respect the fundamental dignity of men and the common biological nature which is at the base of liberty, avoiding manipulations that tend to modify genetic inheritance to create groups of different men at the risk of causing new cases of marginalization in society....
>
> Genetic manipulation becomes arbitrary and unjust when it reduces life to an object, when it forgets that it is dealing

with a human subject, capable of intelligence and freedom, worthy of respect whatever may be their limitations; or when it treats this person in terms of criteria not founded on the integral reality of the human person, at the risk of infringing upon his dignity. In this case, it exposes the individual to the caprice of others, thus depriving him of his autonomy.... (John Paul II 1983; cf. Rodriguez 2000, 36–38)

The Vatican's Congregation for the Doctrine of the Faith also says:

Certain attempts to influence chromosomic or genetic inheritance are not therapeutic but are aimed at producing human beings selected according to sex or other predetermined qualities. These manipulations are contrary to the personal dignity of the human being and his or her integrity and identity. Therefore, in no way can they be justified on the grounds of possible beneficial consequences for future humanity. Every person must be respected for himself: in this consists the dignity and right of every human being from his or her beginning. (CDF 1987, I.6)

Sutton thinks that children may resent others, including their parents, treating them as manufactured products by choosing certain genetic traits for them. Turning children into artifacts involves refusing to accept them as they are, treating them as commodities and objects of manipulation. This depersonalizes them and impoverishes ourselves. It involves "overstepping the boundaries of what we might rightfully do as stewards, but not masters, of our own and our children's earthly natures" (Sutton 1995, 86–87).

The dream of improving human beings by genetic engineering, says Bruce, "is an illusion while, as Jesus declared, it is what is in our hearts which defiles us." "The writer of Psalm 90 observes that even living ten years more than average is no great improvement... There is deliverance 'from this body of death,' but it requires 'a new heavens and a new earth,' the resurrection of the

dead, not merely progressive improvements." "Our ideas of what
we mean by improvement are transient, as for example different
cultures' conceptions in history of the 'ideal' shape for a woman!"
From a Christian point of view, Jesus Christ, the author of our salvation, who came humbly as a servant and was perfected through
suffering (Heb 2:10), is the way to true human improvement. "To
emulate him is our calling, man and woman alike. Paul's ambition
'that Christ may be formed in me' is something very different
from changing our genetics, where we remain uniquely ourselves,
and yet Christ-like. Instead of the uniformity of the ideal, a narrowing of options of our gene pool, there is a rejoicing in diversity, and an expanding of possibilities in Christ" (SRT 1998,
"Moral and Ethical Issues in Gene Therapy"). From a Christian
perspective, true human improvement consists not in being taller
or more intelligent, and so forth, but in growing in loving God
and one another as Jesus loves us (see, e.g., Matt 22:34–40 and
John 13–15; and cf. Walter 2000, 127–28; Keenan 1999; and
Engelhardt 1999).

2.E. Human Cloning

In February 1997 news of the cloned sheep Dolly, the first clone
of a higher adult mammal, provoked much debate worldwide about
the possibility of human cloning and whether or not this should be
allowed. Subsequent reports of Hawaiian scientists producing three
generations of cloned mice and Japanese scientists cloning eight
identical calves from a single adult cow have confirmed the real
possibility of cloning human beings (*Time* 1999, 35; Weiss 1998).
The mechanics and different types of cloning, which have been
explained to some extent above (see 1.D. "Cloning Plants and Animals"), will not be repeated unnecessarily here. As with higher
mammals, several types of cloning with regard to human beings
seem possible: (1) somatic cell nuclear transfer cloning (cf. Dolly);

(2) artificial embryonic splitting, that is, causing identical twins, triplets and so forth, by artificially splitting undifferentiated cells in the early embryo; and (3) cloning certain human cells including stem cells to produce certain human tissues. Today some also distinguish between cloning human embryos for reproductive purposes, that is, to produce a child, and "therapeutic" purposes, that is, the embryo is to be used for research that will hopefully benefit other human beings but not the embryo itself that is destroyed (Flaman 2001, 4–9).

SOMATIC CELL NUCLEAR TRANSFER CLONING

With somatic cell nuclear transfer cloning, the clone would share the same nuclear DNA as the human being from whom it was taken unless random errors were introduced in the cloning process (see Ch. 1.D, par. 2, above). If it worked without producing significant random errors in the clone's DNA, the clone would likely be identical or almost identical physically (consider identical twins), but would be younger, perhaps even by many years. There may be some physical differences in the clone since he or she would be produced from a different ovum, with some differences in its cytoplasm, including mitochondrial DNA. The uterine environment of the clone, perhaps gestated by a different woman, would also not be exactly the same. The clone would not be socialized in exactly the same way either, since even if he or she were raised in the same family, there would be some differences of time and other circumstances.

The clone and the original would be different persons, likely with greater personality differences than identical twins. A cloned human being would be a real person. There is a strong consensus among Jewish, Roman Catholic and Protestant thinkers that "a child created through somatic cell nuclear transfer cloning would still be created in the image of God" (Childress 1997, 11). Such cloning raises certain questions such as who would be the parents of a clone. Theoretically, such cloning would also make human reproduction possible without men. Even if human cloning became widely available, however, I expect that most people would still be drawn by natural desires to procreate in the natural way.

(1) CLONING HUMAN EMBRYOS FOR REPRODUCTIVE PURPOSES

It seems that most people think that reproductive cloning of whole human beings is wrong. Nevertheless, a number of different reasons have been raised as to why this might be done. There also exist a spectrum of ethical and legal views regarding reproductive human cloning. These range from those who think it should be allowed and done for certain reasons, to those who see many problems with it but who do not want to say it would be wrong in every conceivable circumstance, to those who think it would always be immoral and should be legally prohibited.

Dr. Richard Seed, a physicist, wants to be the first to clone a human being. To accomplish this he has been trying to raise 2.5 million dollars. He claims to have a team of several scientists. His argument for doing this includes saying, "God made man in his own image....Therefore, He intended that man should become one with God" by doing the same (*Edmonton Journal* editorial 1998). Seed may not be the first to clone a human being however. The Raelian religious cult, which believes that human cloning is the key to eternal life, has founded Clonaid, a human cloning company (Weiss 2000). In December 1998 a team of scientists in South Korea announced that they have begun work on human cloning. They "claimed to have produced a four-cell human embryo" (Wendy Cole in *Time* 1999, 55). In March 2001, Severino Antinori, an Italian fertility expert, and his U.S. colleague Panayiotis Zavos, announced their intention to offer cloning to infertile couples (BioNews Mar. 12, 2001, "Outrage Over Human Cloning Experiments").

In the 1970s Joseph Fletcher advanced several arguments for cloning human beings that are still raised by some today: "Good reasons in general for cloning are that it avoids genetic diseases, bypasses sterility, predetermines an individual's gender, and preserves family likenesses." Clones could serve as organ donors for each other without risk of rejection. Cloning could also serve the social good, for example, by selectively reproducing individuals with particular traits suited for certain tasks, or to preserve and perpetuate desired or superior genotypes. Fletcher opposes widespread cloning that would reduce genetic variety and undermine survival of the species. He also says some uses of cloning would be immoral, such as reproducing individuals who are distorted functionally. Nevertheless, he argues that sometimes we should clone human beings when biological homogeneity can serve a constructive purpose (Fletcher 1974, 154–56). Other reasons for cloning could include wanting to make a copy of oneself as a form of pseudo-immortality (cf. Rifkin 1998, 218–19). Or, some people may wish to raise a child who is a cloned copy of a famous person. Some argue against strict legal restrictions in a pluralistic society. For example, some speak of reproductive freedom, including a "right" to have a child. Some argue that it is not good to inhibit freedom and progress of research because it rules out not only feared dangers and abuses but also the benefits of such research (cf. *Edmonton Journal* editorial 1998).

Many favor a temporary moratorium on cloning human beings, at least until serious risks of harm can be minimized. Dr. Ian Wilmut, whose team cloned the sheep Dolly, points out that at present cloning is a very inefficient procedure. "The incidence of death among fetuses and offspring produced by cloning is…roughly ten times as high as normal before birth and three times as high after birth in our studies at Roslin." Normal reproduction corrects genetic errors that accumulate in cells and resets the aging clock. We do not know if these occur with cloning. "Research with animals is urgently required to measure the life span and determine the cause of death of animals produced by cloning....An independent body similar to the FDA is now required to assess all the research on cloning" (Wilmut 1999, 52–55). There are signs that Dolly's cells, when she was born, were the same age as the six-year-old ewe from which she was cloned. In April 2000 Robert Lanza and some other scientists, however, reported that they may have figured out a way to reverse the aging process in cells using the cloning technology (Reuters Apr. 28, 2000; Lanza et al. 2000). The recent announcements of a few scientists who plan to attempt reproductive human cloning have met widespread condemnation from other scientists who think the technology is not safe with its high incidence of abnormality and neonatal death in animals (BioNews Mar. 12, 2001; see 1.D, par. 2, above).

In response to Dolly, U.S. President Bill Clinton asked the National Bioethics Advisory Commission to examine the ethical and legal issues raised by the possibility of cloning human beings. In its June 1997 report, this commission concluded that it is morally unacceptable at the present time for anyone in the public or private sector to attempt to create a child using somatic cell nuclear transfer cloning because

> ...current scientific information indicates that this technique is not safe to use in humans at this time....these technologies...are likely to involve unacceptable risks to the fetus and/or potential child. Moreover, in addition to safety concerns, many other serious ethical concerns have been identified, which require much more widespread and careful public deliberation before this technology may be used.

This commission also called for federal legislation to prohibit anyone from attempting to create a child in this way, that such legislation be reviewed after three to five years to decide whether the prohibition continues to be needed, and that no new regulation is required regarding the cloning of human DNA sequences and cell lines (NBAC 1997, 8).

Canada's Royal Commission on New Reproductive Technologies recommended that

> ...some current and potential practices are so harmful and so sharply contravene Canadian ethical and social values that they should not be permitted in Canada on threat of criminal sanction. These include research involving human embryos (zygotes) directed toward development of cloning, ectogenesis, creation of animal/human hybrids...the sale of human eggs, sperm, zygotes, embryos, fetuses or fetal tissue...."
> (RCNRT 1993, 5; cf. MRCC et al. 1998, 9.3)

The Canadian federal government's Proposals for Legislation Governing Assisted Human Reproduction (May 2001), if they become law, would ban the cloning of human beings "because it treats human beings as though they were objects and does not respect the individuality of human beings." A number of international statements, including the World Health Organization Resolutions 50.37 and 51.10 (1998), already ban human cloning (Health Canada 2001, 4–5). The members of the Council of Europe have signed a protocol committing their countries to banning "any intervention seeking to create human beings genetically identical to another human being, whether living or dead" (Catholic News Service 1998). If human beings were ever cloned, this could have many legal implications including the development of a whole new area of litigation. For example, some cloned human beings, who were damaged in the process or perhaps simply not happy with their genetic endowments, could file lawsuits against their makers.

Some ethicists and other people see many problems with cloning human beings but do not want to say that it would be wrong in every conceivable circumstance. Although Tim Caulfield, research director of the University of Alberta's Health Law Institute, acknowledges that there are many health, ethical and safety concerns associated with cloning human beings, he sees nothing inherently wrong with this. He favors regulatory means rather than criminal prohibitory laws which he thinks give legitimacy to the reductionist view that human beings are no more than the sum of their genes (Thorne 2001).

A number of Protestant, Jewish and secular thinkers "worry about inappropriate uses or abuses of human cloning." They view it as morally neutral or morally problematic, "but not intrinsically wrong." Some think cloning human beings can only be justified for certain reasons such as a person or couple has no other means to reproduce or to avoid having a child with a genetic disease carried by one spouse. A number of ethicists, religious organizations, and others, however, have concluded that cloning human beings would never be ethical.

> Some thinkers, especially but not only in the Roman Catholic tradition, hold that cloning humans is wrong in and of itself (intrinsically wrong), and that it would thus be wrong under any conceivable circumstances. Any use would violate human dignity, the natural law, the natural order, or some other fundamental principle or value.... (Childress 1997, 10)

The Church of Scotland considers cloning human beings "ethically unacceptable as a matter of principle...a violation of the basic dignity and uniqueness of each human being made in God's image, of what God has given to that individual [and] to no one else." The nature of cloning is that of "an instrumental use of both the clone and the one cloned as means to an end, for someone else's benefit. This represents unacceptable human abuse, and a potential for exploitation which should be outlawed worldwide" (SRT 1998, "Cloning Animals and Humans").

The Vatican's Congregation for the Doctrine of the Faith teaches that "attempts...for obtaining a human being without any connection with sexuality through 'twin fission,' cloning or parthenogenesis are to be considered contrary to the moral law, since they are in opposition to the dignity both of human procreation and of the conjugal union" (CDF 1987, I.6). Bishop Elio Sgreccia, the Vatican's leading expert on medical ethics, says, "Human cloning would violate human dignity, the dignity of marriage and the very principle of human equality." Human equality would not allow such a "total domination over the human being, who would be manufactured and reproduced." One fear of cloning is its potential use in creating a "super race" of people with specific characteristics (Gonzalez 1997, 1; cf. Thavis 1999, 5). Richard Doerflinger, an adviser to the U.S. bishops, says cloning "is not a worthy way to bring a human being into the world. Children have a right to have real parents, and to be conceived as the fruit of marital love between husband and wife." Children "are not products we can manufacture to our specifications" (Gonzalez 1997, 3). In practice, cloning human beings would also involve other immoral practices such as discarding "defective," "abnormal" and "unwanted" embryos and carrying out non-therapeutic experiments on some or all of them (cf. CDF 1987, I.4–6 and II.5).

Varga thinks there may be some good uses for cell fusion, cloning, and so forth, regarding plants and animals, but thinks there is no valid reason for attempting these on humans. They would violate some fundamental values concerning human procreation and would be dehumanizing. Producing a human clone would treat this person as an object, not a person, a mere means for others' goals or wishes (Varga 1984, Ch. 6).

Dr. Ian Wilmut, whose team cloned the sheep Dolly, discusses possible motives for reproductive human cloning, for example: to overcome an infertility problem; to make "a copy of one partner in a homosexual relationship or of a single parent"; and to try to bring back a relative such as a child tragically killed. Concerning the last case he notes that the clone would be a different person. It is likely that the clone would be expected to be the same as the lost relative. This would be placing unnatural and unfair expectations on him or her. In making a "copy" of a living person, how would the clone feel seeing his or her physical future ahead of him or her? Would the original be even more inclined to impose expectations on the cloned child than the average parent? Wilmut concludes that "every child should be wanted for itself, as an individual. In making a copy of oneself or some famous person, a parent is deliberately specifying the way he or she wishes the child to develop." In recent years much emphasis has been placed on the right of individuals to reproduce in ways that they wish. "There is a greater need to consider the interests of the child and to reject cloning" (Wilmut 1999, 52–54).

Along similar lines, Daniel Callahan says:

> Nowhere has anyone suggested that cloning would advance the cause of children....It has been one of the enduring failures of the reproductive rights movement that it has...constantly dissociated the needs of children and the desires of would-be parents. Instead of taking the high road and focusing on what children require for a good life...the reproductive rights movement consistently drifts toward a lower standard....In other words, if anything now goes, then it would be an offense to procreative rights not to extend that permissive sanction to human cloning. (Callahan 1997, 19; cf. Kaveny 1999, 135–40)

Callahan challenges such individualism.

Although couples who cannot have children genetically related to them by moral means may understandably suffer, no one has a right to have a child. Children should be accepted as a gift of God and loved unconditionally as God loves. Anyone, whether biologically fertile or not, can still bear much spiritual fruit that will last by living in union with God (cf. John 15). The Congregation for the Doctrine of the Faith points out that infertile couples can still serve "the life of the human person" in various ways, for example, by "adoption, various forms of educational work, and assistance to other families and to poor or handicapped children" (CDF 1987, II.8).

In 1993 George Washington University researchers cloned human embryos by artificial embryo splitting and nurtured them in a Petri dish for several days. This project provoked "protests from ethicists, politicians and critics of genetic engineering" (*Time* 1999, 34). Although identical twinning by natural causes involves natural "cloning," it is not ethical for us to do everything that happens in physical nature. For instance, a natural flood killing many people does not justify humans causing a flood to kill many people. Many of the arguments both for and against somatic cell nuclear transfer cloning could be applied to this type of cloning as well.

(2) CLONING HUMAN EMBRYOS FOR "THERAPEUTIC" PURPOSES

Some advocate cloning human embryos not for reproductive but for "therapeutic" purposes. For example, some argue in favor of research to produce embryonic clones from healthy cells of a patient with Parkinson's disease, burn victims, leukemia and so forth, to produce tissues including bone marrow for transplant that would incur no danger of rejection unlike tissue from an unrelated donor (Nash 1998; cf. Klotzko 1997, 436–37). Not unrelated to such research, in 1998 some scientists reported having removed embryonic stem cells from human blastocysts (about 140 cell stage embryos) and getting them to differentiate into certain types of body cells. Some hope that such research will lead to the production of various tissues not only for transplant purposes, for example, to replace brain cells and patch heart muscle, but also to provide normal human tissues for testing the toxicity of new drugs (Lemonick 1998; Geron 1999).

In 1997 it was also reported that some British scientists had created "a frog embryo without a head" by manipulating certain genes to suppress development of the tadpole's head, trunk and tail. Combined with human cloning, the technique "may lead to the production of headless human clones to grow organs and tissue for transplant." Embryologist Jonathan Slack says, "Instead of growing an intact embryo, you could genetically reprogram the embryo to suppress growth in all the parts of the body except the bits you want, plus a heart and blood circulation." Some argue that such organisms would not be normal embryos and human beings, so no one would be harmed. One critic, Professor Andrew Linzey, however, says, "It is morally regressive to create a mutant form of life" (The Associated Press 1997).

The Federal Government of Canada's (May 2001) Proposals for Legislation Governing Assisted Human Reproduction, if they become law, would prohibit "therapeutic cloning" in humans. The Overview document notes that such cloning "in animals has raised many health and safety concerns" and it is, therefore, "too risky to proceed" with humans. It recommends research on "stem cells taken from existing human embryos" and notes that there is "an international consensus that limits research to the first 14 days of embryonic development" (Health Canada 2001, 5; cf. Canadian Institute of Health Research 2001). Canada's proposed legislation on this topic is more restrictive than that of the United Kingdom. On January 22, 2001, the House of Lords approved a controversial law that will allow British scientists to clone human embryos for medical research (The Associated Press London 2001).

On August 9, 2001, United States President George W. Bush, after hearing representations from various sides, announced that he would "authorize federal funds for embryonic stem-cell research involving only the 60 or so existing stem-cell lines already developed by scientists, because in those cases 'the life-and death decision has already been made.'" His intention was not to provide "taxpayer funding that would sanction or encourage further destruction of human embryos." He expressed his strong opposition to human cloning and his support for "aggressive federal funding of research on umbilical cord, placenta, adult and animal stem cells." Responses to his announcement ranged from those who praised his decision, to those who considered it too restrictive, to those who said it promotes complicity in evil since research on stem-cell lines derived from embryos would benefit those who originally destroyed the embryos to obtain these stem cells. President Bush also announced his plans to set up a council to recommend appropriate guidelines and to monitor stem cell research (Frazier O'Brien 2001. Cf. BioNews Aug. 13, 2001; and Filteau 2001).

Today there is a lot of hype regarding research on cloning human embryos for "therapeutic" purposes and research on embryonic stem cells. A couple of facts, however, should be kept in mind to keep this in perspective. As noted above (1.D, par. 2), it seems that random errors in the clone's DNA often occur in the cloning process. Many cloned animals suffer from a variety of abnormalities. If such errors often occur in cloning animal embryos, they are likely to occur in cloning human embryos, whether for reproductive or "therapeutic" purposes. Any cells, tissues or organs produced from such embryos would carry the same errors with potential problems. It has also been recently reported that the "first full trial to treat Parkinson's disease using transplanted fetal brain cells has produced disappointing results, with serious side effects occurring in some patients" (BioNews Mar. 3, 2001; cf. Doerflinger 1999). These are only a couple of the serious technical problems that would need to be overcome to achieve the goals many hope for from such research.

From an ethical perspective, the results of such research are not the only thing that needs to be considered. While some of the "goals" of such proposals may be good, that is, to provide benefits for many people, the "means" also need careful ethical evaluation. First of all, it needs to be kept in mind that the human embryo (or zygote or fetus), whether it results from normal in vivo fertilization or in vitro fertilization or cloning, is a human being. It should always be treated as a person with the basic rights of a person, including the right to life (see 2.A.1 above under "Abortion"). In the research we are considering here, the intention is not to benefit the embryonic human being. It is not "therapeutic" for him or her.

Rather, it involves treating him or her as a mere means to others' good, as an object to be used, exploited, manipulated and/or destroyed. This is clearly contrary to his or her great fundamental dignity which is equal to that of other human beings. Secondly, the means of producing such human beings by cloning is immoral in itself. Like in vitro fertilization, cloning dissociates human procreation from its proper context, a fruit of the conjugal act within a loving marriage. It also "establishes the domination of technology over the origin and destiny of the human person" which is contrary to the dignity and equality common to embryonic human beings and other human beings (CDF 1987, II.5).

Moreover, it should be noted that many, perhaps even all or more, of the benefits that some hope for from research on stem cells obtained from human embryos may become available by alternative means. These include using pluripotent stem cells from adult tissues such as skin, blood, bone marrow, and fat, or from blood harvested from the placenta and umbilical cord of newborn infants. "For example, functional genes for...inherited diseases may be amenable to gene therapy using cord blood stem cells as the vehicle" (Stephenson 1995, 1814). Recently, a team of American scientists found a way to reprogram easily obtainable human fat stem cells to produce various other tissue types. Adam Katz, a team member from the University of Pittsburgh, said that "the potential use of fat cells could make the use of controversial fetal or embryonic stem cells obsolete. It would also have the added benefit of being a genetic match to the person who was treated with stem cells—or, in the future, tissues cultivated from them—so the problem of tissue transplant rejection may be overcome" (BioNews Apr. 17, 2001. See also USCC 2000; and The Associated Press 2000). Research and transplants involving stem cells from human cord blood or adult tissues to be ethical would require the free and informed consent of the donor or guardian, and so forth, but they would not involve the immoral exploitation, manipulation and destruction of embryonic human beings. Along these lines, Pope John Paul II says:

Methods that fail to respect the dignity and value of the person must always be avoided. I am thinking in particular of attempts at human cloning with a view to obtaining organs for transplants: these techniques, insofar as they involve the manipulation and destruction of human embryos, are not morally acceptable, even when their proposed goal is good in itself. Science itself points to other forms of *therapeutic intervention* which would not involve cloning or the use of embryonic cells, but rather would make use of stem cells taken from adults. This is the direction that research must follow if it wishes to respect the dignity of each and every human being, even at the embryonic stage. (John Paul II 2000, 2)

2.F. Eugenics

The term *eugenic* means "well-born." Eugenics involves improving the genetic makeup of a population by human intervention. "Negative eugenics" tries to reduce genetic defects. "Positive eugenics" tries to increase desirable genetic traits (Varga 1984, 75–76; Rodriguez 1998, 74). Some writers today distinguish the "old eugenics" movement and the "new eugenics."

The old eugenics movement grew rapidly in the early twentieth century. Based on scientific views of the time regarding evolution and genetics it gained the support of many leading scientists, politicians and much of the public in many countries, including England, Germany, the United States and Canada. Many feared that medicine was keeping alive "unfit" people to reproduce their kind, resulting in an increase of poverty, crime and other social problems. Eugenics was seen as the way to solve such problems. Although some promoted positive eugenics by more breeding of the "fit," one of the main means of negative eugenics practiced in many countries was legalized involuntary sterilization of the mentally and physically "unfit." Eugenics linked to certain racist ideas influenced immigration policies in the United States. Such ideas were also used in Nazi Germany to "justify" not only the killing of innocent disabled people but many healthy people as well. Negative reaction to these latter atrocities was one of the major factors in the decline of the eugenics movement after World War II. In hindsight this older eugenics movement is seen to have been based on simplistic views of genetics and solving social problems, as well as genetic reductionism and prejudice (for more details see the Introduction above; Arthur Dyck in Kilner et al. 1997, 25–30; Paul Gray in *Time* 1999, 62–63; Hubbard and Wald 1993, Ch. 2).

Varga says that the main reasons given for eugenic involuntary sterilization were: (1) "the common good demands the prevention of the birth of defective offspring who are a burden to society"; and (2) those who "cannot fulfill the basic duties of parenthood... should not be allowed to reproduce." He, however, argues that

> eugenic sterilization...is not necessary for the prevention of any great evil threatening society. Persons with a low I.Q. or those who are physically defective, or alcoholics, can have very healthy and bright offspring, as many such cases have been recorded in history. Criminal behavior is not transmitted by genes to the offspring. The state does not have a right over the bodies of innocent citizens. Societies and governments are formed to protect the rights of the individuals and not to take them away. (Varga 1984, 81)

He also argues that sterilizing criminals is not justified and would hardly deter a prospective criminal (Varga 1984, 79–84. See also LRCC 1979 for an overview of arguments raised for and against involuntary sterilization).

In the United States a few states have procedures to allow the mentally handicapped to be voluntarily sterilized while protecting them against unnecessary or involuntary sterilization (LRCC 1979, 85–88). In "Eve v. Mrs. E" the Supreme Court of Canada ruled against non-therapeutic involuntary sterilization. The judgment warns against "abuse of the mentally incompetent" and says in part that "the onus of proving the need for the procedure [sterilization of the incompetent] is on those who seek to have it performed" (Supreme Court of Canada 1986, 418). In a number of places some victims of involuntary sterilization are now receiving substantial monetary compensation for the irreversible damages done to them. The documentary, *The Sterilization of Leilani Muir,* illustrates such a case (see NFB 1996).

Jean Vanier, the founder of L'Arche, has been living and working with mentally handicapped people since 1964. With regard to involuntary sterilization of the mentally handicapped he concludes, "It is a serious injustice to so mutilate someone, especially when it is done without even asking the person's permission" (Vanier 1985, 151). He says some parents or guardians are more worried that a handicapped woman might conceive a child than they are concerned to protect her from being sexually abused. Not only the handicapped but also their care givers, however, need support and solidarity from other families and the Christian community. Vanier criticizes those who advocate sexual permissiveness for the handicapped. This does not help them to develop their capacities for love and relationship, but risks imprisoning them in a search for pleasure that finally isolates them more than ever. While he is aware that severely mentally handicapped people are not able to responsibly marry and procreate, he thinks that some mildly mentally handicapped people are capable of marrying and parenting with some help from others. Some people in our society see the disabled as the least valuable members of society. Vanier, however, says their greater needs call others to a greater love. Since growing in love is what is most important from a Christian perspective, the disabled can be seen as the most important members of a community. Vanier considers human pride to be the greatest handicap since it is the greatest obstacle to love (Vanier 1985, Chs. 5–8).

Catholic teaching considers contraceptive sterilization, whether involuntary or voluntary, to be intrinsically disordered. One of the first world leaders to condemn eugenic sterilization was Pope Pius

XI. In his 1930 encyclical on Christian marriage, among other things, he describes legislation in favor of involuntary eugenic sterilization as civil authority arrogating "to itself a power over a faculty that it never had and can never legitimately possess." Those who act in this way lose sight of the fact that human beings "are begotten not for the earth and for time, but for Heaven and eternity." Christian teaching and human reason makes clear that individuals themselves also "are not free to destroy or mutilate their members, or in any other way render themselves unfit for their natural functions, except when no other provision can be made for the good of the whole body." Contraception and contraceptive sterilization are against the law of God and nature. Abortion, also for eugenic "indications," is unthinkable murder of the innocent (Pius XI 1930, 27–36). Catholic teaching today continues to hold that no reason can justify direct contraception, sterilization and abortion, but that married couples can use Natural Family Planning for just reasons (see Paul VI 1968; John Paul II 1981, nn. 28–35; as well as Ch. 2.A.4 above). Concerning this issue, the *Catechism of the Catholic Church* teaches in part: "Except when performed for strictly therapeutic medical reasons, directly intended...*sterilizations* performed on innocent persons are against the moral law" (CCC 1999, n. 2297; cf. USCC 1994, n. 53; and CHAC 2000, 13 and 40).

Today some speak of a "new eugenics" related to the new genetic engineering tools. For example, prenatal diagnosis with selective abortion and preimplantation diagnosis with the discarding of "abnormal" embryos involves negative eugenics. So would germ-line gene therapy that would affect any offspring. Somatic gene therapy, however, would not involve eugenics since any changes would not affect offspring. Genetic design and enhancement that affects the germ-line would involve positive eugenics. So would selecting embryos with desirable genetic traits for implantation, as well as selecting sperm or ova with desirable genetic traits for artificial insemination and/or in vitro fertilization procedures. Cloning human beings with desirable or "superior" genetic traits would also involve positive eugenics (see, e.g., Hubbard and Wald 1993, Ch. 3; Rodriguez 1998, 77–81; and Arthur Dyck in Kilner et al. 1997, 30–37). Since we have already considered the ethics of these methods (see 2.A-E above), we will limit our discussion here to a few other considerations.

Some enthusiasts of eugenics today are still concerned that modern medicine, by keeping more people alive to reproduce, is increasing the load of defective genes in the human gene pool and upsetting the ecological balance. The consensus of the best medical and genetic opinion, however, is that "whatever genetic deterioration is occurring as a result of decreased natural selection is so slow as to be insignificant…" (Lappe as cited in Ashley and O'Rourke 1997, 251). Trying to eliminate disabilities by negative eugenics is an unrealistic goal, since only a small percent of disabilities are from birth. Most are due to accidents and illnesses later in life (CBC 1992). Since the same persons carry both good and bad genetic traits, trying to eliminate genetic defects from the human gene pool by negative eugenics would eliminate many good genetic traits as well (Ashley and O'Rourke 1997, 250–52). In fact, since everyone of us has some genetic defects, where would we stop? In any case, respecting the principle of free and informed consent requires that any decisions with eugenic effects be both voluntary and well-informed (cf. Ch. 2.B above).

Rifkin points out that while the old eugenics involved government control and was spurred by political ideology, fear and hate, the new eugenics is being spurred by market forces and consumer desire (Rifkin 1998, 128). Eugenics today is being driven by many parents not wanting an "abnormal" child or wanting only a normal, healthy and/or superior child. The cumulative effect of the free workings of parental desire and choice can achieve the same results as a state-organized eugenics program that aims at reducing genetic disease in the population and related societal costs. According to Roy, Williams and Dickens, however, some critics today argue that "leaving all decisions to the discretion of parents…indicates the low value our society places upon those with genetic disorders and handicaps." They say that we need to promote tolerance for differences to prevent "such tragic eugenic devaluation of human beings" (Roy et al. 1994, 188–89; cf. Robert Wright in *Time* 1999, 51; CBC 1992). I agree.

Discussion Questions

1. Tests show a pregnant mother is carrying a child with an inherited disease and is highly likely to develop an associated deafness. Would you recommend termination? If yes, you have just aborted Beethoven (cf. Harris 1992, 179). If tests indicate that a human fetus probably has a certain genetic disorder, do you think that the woman or couple should talk with people who have this disorder? (See 2.A.1 and 2.B above.)

2. Should an insurance company be able to have access to a client or prospective client's genetic information? Should they be able to refuse coverage or be able to charge higher premiums based on such information? Should someone who is presymptomatic but has a genetic disease such as Huntington's disease be able to buy more health or life insurance than normal without letting the insurer know? Should an employer be able to have access to an employee's or a prospective employee's genetic information? Should they be able to make hiring or firing decisions based on such information? (See 2.B above.)

3. If you knew you were a carrier for a serious genetic disorder would you ask a prospective marriage partner to be tested before agreeing to get married? (See 2.A.4 above.)

4. If you loved someone and otherwise wanted to marry him or her, but genetic tests indicated there was a 25% chance that your children would have a certain genetic disorder would

you still marry him or her? Would a lower (e.g., 5%) or higher (e.g., 50%) chance make any difference? Would the severity of the disorder make any difference? (See 2.A.4 above.)

5. You and your spouse each has a nephew with the same genetic disorder. Would you take part in a genetic screening program before conception occurs? What criteria would you use to determine whether or not you will have children? (Adapted from Ashley and O'Rourke 1994, 188.)

6. If you were already married to someone would a 5%, 25% or 50% chance of passing a genetic disorder to your children influence your family planning decisions? Would the severity of the disorder make any difference (consider, e.g., Down's syndrome, cystic fibrosis, Huntington's disease)?

7. If you were to choose a career as a genetic counselor, what are some difficult ethical issues that you would likely face? Should a counselor ever divulge a person's genetic information to third parties? Is it possible for a counselor to be completely "neutral" or "non-directive"? Should a counselor always share the whole "truth" with a client, even if the possible harm of such sharing may outweigh the benefits? Should a counselor only provide information? Should a counselor provide emotional support? What should a counselor do if she or he cannot in good conscience support her or his client's plans or decision, e.g., to terminate a pregnancy because the couple does not want a girl? What kind of role, if any, can counselors have in helping clients make sound ethical decisions? (See 2.B above, as well as other parts of this book.)

8. A research scientist from the United States seeks to cure a genetic defect in a native of Africa by means of recombinant DNA (gene splicing) that supplements a defective gene in the genotype of the patient. A federal agency declares his efforts unethical and cancels his research funds. Would this involve somatic or germ-line gene therapy? When and under what

conditions will such research be ethically acceptable? (Adapted from Ashley and O'Rourke 1994, 188; see 2.C above.)

9. If you were designing a "new" human being, what changes in design and function, if any, do you think would improve human life? Consider also genetically modifying some human beings to live in a different environment, e.g., in outer space or on another planet. (Adapted from Ashley and O'Rourke 1994, 187; see 2.D above.)

10. If you were offered the chance to have a clone of yourself made (e.g., by Dr. Seed or Dr. Antinori), how would you respond? Should anyone, including infertile couples, homosexuals and single people, be allowed to reproduce by whatever means they wish, including cloning? What form of human procreation and parenting is in the best interests of children? (See 2.E.1 above.)

11. Discuss the ethics of cloning human embryos to obtain embryonic stem cells for research that many hope will lead to various cures. Is this using an evil means for a good end? Should such research be banned with emphasis being put rather on research involving stem cells obtained from adults or umbilical cord blood? (See 2.E.2 above.)

12. Should single women or men or married people, e.g., mentally disabled or sexually irresponsible persons, ever be sterilized without their consent? (See 2.F above.)

Chapter Three

Various Views of Plant, Animal and Human Life

In Chapters 1 and 2 we considered some different arguments and conclusions regarding a number of specific issues related to the genetic engineering of plants, animals and human beings. Underlying these different arguments and conclusions are various views of plant, animal and human life.

Rifkin says the new biotechnologies with clones, chimeras and transgenic animals poignantly raise the question of how we should view our fellow species and our own (Rifkin 1998, 103). He speaks of two kinds of science today that each view and approach biological organisms and nature differently. Many molecular biologists and geneticists, who are seeking to reprogram the genetic components of life, have a fragmentary view of life. As heirs to the Baconian tradition of science, they take a reductionist, detached approach to nature. They seek to master nature and put it in the service of humankind. Francis Bacon saw nature as at fault for human miseries. He sought knowledge to exercise power over nature. His view reduced nature's value to its usefulness for us (Allen Verhey in Kilner et al. 1997, 62–63). Today there are also others in the field of biology who take a more integrative and systematic approach to nature.

They seek to enhance existing relationships and preserve ecological diversity. Many ecological scientists think the preservation of species is a moral imperative. These different views or approaches to life lead to different practices in agriculture and medicine. Rifkin thinks these two approaches should complement each other (Rifkin 1998, 227–29).

Our cosmologies are based in the real world, but only that small portion of the real world where society and nature interact. They are socially biased and used to legitimize the way individuals and institutions do things, that is, as a reflection of the "natural order of things." For example, medieval society was hierarchically organized. Related to this, medieval cosmology (e.g., Aquinas) viewed all of reality as hierarchical. Darwin lived in the industrial or machine age. The English culture of his day was influenced by capitalism and colonization. Related to this the cosmology of Darwinism includes evolution, competition and survival of the fittest, and views life as complex machines. Today a different view of nature is emerging. It is related to process philosophy, cybernetics and a network-based global economy. Living organisms are seen as dynamic self-organizing processes that are continually adapting with negative and positive feedback. Evolution in this view is not seen merely as random and passive. Nature is cast in the image of the computer and the language of physics, chemistry, mathematics and the information sciences. This view of life legitimizes genetic engineering. Darwin's mechanical conception of living beings robbed them of intrinsic value and any sacred qualities. Their value was seen in terms of their utility. Viewing life as information eliminates the idea of species integrity. With this view there is no longer any question of sacredness or specialness, no longer any recognizable boundaries to respect. Structure, essences and substance are abandoned. Everything is seen as pure activity and process (Rifkin 1998, Ch. 7; cf. Moltmann 1985, 26–27; and Ashley 1985).

"The problem, once again, is that in our cosmologies we inflate the tiny aspect of nature's reality that we are manipulating at a moment in time into a universal cosmology and then claim that all of nature operates in a manner that is congenial with the way we are operating." The concept of knowledge is being reduced to information. In our nanosecond culture where everything changes so fast, change is honored as the only timeless truth. The idea of an "objective" reality is giving way to the idea of "perspectives" of reality, the idea of "permanent truths" is giving way to "useful models" in postmodernism (Rifkin 1998, 216–21). In *Fides et Ratio,* Pope John Paul II provides a balanced response to such contemporary views. Among other things, he affirms the existence of "universal truths" (John Paul II, 1998).

Today some see us as having a momentous responsibility as the architects of nature, the creators of life. Bioengineering is seen as the next stage in the evolutionary process. Life, long viewed as God's handiwork, is now being "reimagined as an artistic medium with untold possibilities." This view, however, involves a misappropriation of technics, which enlarge human power, with art, which involves a deep communion with the outside world and is an expression of love. We "mistakenly think of the new technological manipulation as a creative act, when in reality it is merely a set of choices purchased in the marketplace…the new genetic technologies grant us a godlike power…the greatest shopping experience of all time" (Rifkin 1998, 222–26).

With regard to different views of life today, one often encounters different views with regard to animals in particular. While a variety of animals and animal products have long been used for human food and clothing, a number of people today are turning to vegetarianism. With regard to using animals in research, there exist conflicting views. Some animal rights activists argue that to treat animals any differently than members of our own species is unfair. Many, however, argue that using animals in research that does not benefit them is necessary to reduce risks of harm to human beings. The suffering of animals used in research, however, should be kept to a minimum (cf. Roy et al. 1994, 333–34). With regard to different views of animals consider, for example, also different religious traditions, including the "sacred cow" in Hinduism. In 1995 a number of groups of indigenous people, in a declaration on the Human Genome Diversity Project, expressed their view that creation is sacred. In defense of the sacred harmony of nature they reject all genetic technologies "which manipulate and change the fundamental core and identity of any life form" (Indigenous Peoples 1995).

With regard to different views of life in a pluralistic world, we can ask: What is the place or contribution of beliefs and religious perspectives? In particular, what can a more general Christian and a more specific Catholic perspective offer to a discussion of genetic engineering? Many non-Christians appreciate the concerns and insights that have been raised by Christians. Not all non-Christians, however, use theological language or include God in their perspective (cf. Rollinson 1999; and Ashley 1985, Ch. 3). The natural and social sciences cannot provide us with answers to ultimate questions such as the meaning of life. Deane-Drummond says the failure of science to provide us "with any effective answers to complex environmental issues" and applied biotechnology "is occasion enough to widen the debate to include other disciplines" including theology, philosophy and ethics. "A theological critique requires a radical change of attitude in formulating the goals of genetic engineering from one based on consumerism and the individual pursuit of happiness to a more community-based view that includes respect for the whole environment." She points out that a theological approach "does not necessarily ban all genetic engineering, but seeks to transform it so that it more clearly represents a fully human enterprise" (Deane-Drummond 1995, 318–21; cf. John Paul II's promotion of an "integral humanism," 1995a, 84). Deane-Drummond also maintains that "while the dialogue between different faiths is important in contributing to the practical task of policy making in genetic engineering, each faith needs to become aware of its own distinctive contribution. A lowest common denominator approach is unlikely to yield the promised fruit and more likely to raise false hopes" (Deane-Drummond 1995, 322). While welcoming the contributions of those of other faiths, in the following we will consider some of the contributions which a Christian perspective can offer to our topic of genetic engineering. Catholic theology and teaching affirm the unity of all truth, whether discovered by us or revealed to us by God. Although we do not have all the answers, there cannot be a real contradiction between the true conclusions of scientists, philosophers and theologians (see, e.g., Ashley 1985; John Paul II 1998; and Polkinghorne 1998, a scientist and an Anglican priest).

A Christian Perspective

The Bible affirms the existence of one infinitely good, loving, intelligent and personal God who created everything else out of nothing. In a literary form and language appropriate to the time, Genesis 1 speaks of the goodness of God's creation, including the goodness of plants, animals and human beings. The goodness, order and integrity of creation, including the interrelationships of creatures, reflects the goodness and wisdom of God. Human beings are unique in the visible world. Male and female, they are created in the "image of God" and commissioned to "subdue" or have "dominion" over the earth. This "dominion" was to be exercised in wisdom and love, to meet human needs and to give glory to God (cf. CCC 1999, nn. 279–84; John Paul II 1989, n. 4; and Walter 2000, 124–29). Deane-Drummond says the exercise of our "dominion over creation is qualified by the essence of the relationship between Creator and creation as one of loving involvement.…God's love for all creation demands a respect for the interests of all creatures." She says the engineering of animals to be more passive in crowded conditions, for example, seems to be "an unacceptable violation of that creature's interests." She argues for "protection of the interests of the species…as long as it is set in the context of the *interests* of global ecology and issues of justice related to the human community" (Deane-Drummond 1995, 314–19).

Pope John Paul II notes that "...*the aesthetic value of creation cannot be overlooked.* Our very contact with nature has a deep restorative power; contemplation of its magnificence imparts peace and serenity. The Bible speaks again and again of the goodness and beauty of creation, which is called to glorify God"(John Paul II 1989, n. 14). The Church of Scotland speaks of the sheer diversity of creation as a cause of praise to its Creator:"We may use animals to an extent, but we need to remind ourselves that they are firstly God's creatures, to whom we may not do everything we like" (SRT 1997,"General Assembly Report—Cloning Animals and Humans"). Moltmann points out that understanding the world as God's creation means that "it remains his property" to be "accepted as a loan and administered as a trust" by us (Moltmann 1985, 30–31). Among other things, such a view can help to promote the just sharing of the goods of creation with all human beings as are all God's children.

In 1979 Pope John Paul II proclaimed St. Francis of Assisi the patron saint of those who promote ecology, and said that St. Francis offers

> an example of genuine and deep respect for the integrity of creation. As a friend of the poor who was loved by God's creatures, Saint Francis invited all of creation—animals, plants, natural forces, even Brother Sun and Sister Moon—to give honor and praise to the Lord. The poor man of Assisi gives us striking witness that when we are at peace with God we are better able to devote ourselves to building up that peace with all creation which is inseparable from peace among all peoples. (John Paul II 1989, n. 16)

Created in God's image, human beings have a special and equal dignity. Our equality calls for a fair distribution of goods. Solidarity and sharing are indispensable (John Paul II 1995a, 83). With regard to genetic engineering and questions of human justice, Deane-Drummond says, "A Christian theological perspective would insist on examining the long-term consequences to poorer nations and communities" (Deane-Drummond 1995, 320).

Created in God's image we human beings are also "far more than the sum of our DNA complement" (SRT 1998, "Moral and Ethical Issues in Gene Therapy"). "In his mystery, man goes beyond the sum of his biological characteristics. He is a fundamental unit, in which the biological cannot be separated from the spiritual, family and social dimensions without incurring the serious risk of suppressing the person's very nature..." (John Paul II 1995a, 82; cf. Rollinson 1999). Human beings have a body and spiritual soul (cf. Matt 10:28; CCC 1999, nn. 362–68). Through our bodies we are profoundly related to the physical universe and the earth's ecosystem. Since each of us has a spiritual soul we can have an intimate personal relationship with God who is Spirit (cf. John 4:24). In contemporary language we can speak of a number of levels of human needs and dimensions of the human person: biological, psychological, social, ethical and spiritual. All of these affect human personality (cf. Ashley and O'Rourke 1994, Chs. 1–2).

Pope John Paul II thinks that genome research will enable us to better understand ourselves, in particular, distinguishing genetic influences "from those stemming from the natural and cultural surroundings and those associated with the individual's own experience. In addition, by shedding light on the web of influences within which man exercises his freedom, we will arrive at a clearer understanding of this mysterious reality." Pope John Paul II also says that discoveries of the complexity of the molecular structure can invite us "to wonder about the First Cause, about the One who is the origin of all existence and who has secretly fashioned each one of us (cf. Ps 139:15; Prov 24:12)" (John Paul II 1995a, 81–83). Deane-Drummond thinks that the "traditional understanding of God as transcendent yet immanent in creation provides a way through the current vogue of 'naturalism' into a more realistic and fruitful dialogue with science" (Deane-Drummond 1995, 323). Moltmann points out that the biblical theocentric view can help human beings to understand themselves as members of "the community of creation." This can free us "from the modern anthropocentric view of the world" and help us to find the wisdom to deal with creation and the ecological crisis (Moltmann 1985, 31; cf. Gustafson 1984).

In our age of specialization it is easy to fall into reductionist views and fail to appreciate the mystery of life, of persons and of God. Having an integral holistic vision helps us to respond to specific questions, including those raised by genetic engineering, more adequately. Dr. Donald Bruce says genetics should be evaluated not merely in material and economic terms, but seen "within the wider framework of divine and human relationships." Our relationships with God, ourselves, other human beings and the rest of God's created order involve moral limits in order for us to give glory to God, responsibly meet human needs and be good stewards. "Scripture, history and prudence all indicate the need to limit our creativity— that 'can' does not imply 'ought.'" We are finite and need to keep in mind our limits and failings. We need a proper sense of humility and wonder. Genetics is still a relatively young science. Prudence and caution are in order (SRT 1998, "Moral and Ethical Issues in Gene Therapy"). In line with the above, we can also consider Ashley and O'Rourke's Principle of Stewardship and Creativity:

> The gifts of multidimensional human nature and its natural environment should be used with profound respect for their intrinsic teleology. The gift of human creativity especially should be used to cultivate nature and environment with a care set by the limits of our actual knowledge and the risks of destroying these gifts. (Ashley and O'Rourke 1997, 202)

God's creation is not the only relevant Christian teaching with regard to our topic of genetic engineering. To have an integral vision, creation needs to be understood together with a number of other biblical and Christian theological themes such as sin, redemption and the incarnation. Each of these will only be touched on here briefly. Human sin involves freely choosing to go against God's plan, a failure on our part to love God, ourselves and the rest of God's creation properly. Sin not only alienates us from God, but also from ourselves and the rest of creation. Regarding human sin, "genetics is no more immune from our perverse ability to turn whatever we discover to greedy, abusive and exploitative ends than any other technology" (SRT 1998, "Moral and Ethical Issues in Gene Therapy").

God does not violate human freedom and allows us to sin. In his great love and mercy for us, however, God wants to save or redeem us from sin and all its negative consequences. God's redeeming love, if we freely cooperate with it, reconciles us with God, ourselves and the rest of creation. It restores harmonious relationships. According to a Christian perspective, our complete redemption will also include the resurrection of our bodies, our sharing fully in God's eternal life, love and happiness, and a new transformed heaven and earth. This will all be much better than we can now imagine or dream. Redemption does not mean that we will not suffer in this life or die. All people suffer at times in their life, whether poor or wealthy, ill or healthy, having a genetically based disease or not. Human suffering, however, can have redemptive value or meaning. This is true not only regarding the suffering of Jesus but also regarding the suffering of each one of us (see, e.g., Col 1:24). The Apostle Paul affirms that if we love God, he will work out everything for our good (Rom 8:28). The "everything" here includes not only the good and enjoyable things in our lives but also the bad, the difficult, indeed all our sufferings. Among other things, this can include the extra difficulties of raising a child with disabilities or enduring the sufferings of a genetic disease oneself. Jesus, who suffered in many ways in his life on earth, including a cruel death on the cross, is a good model for us in this regard. Jesus loved God through all this. If we consider not only Jesus' suffering and death but also his resurrection and ascension into glory, we can realize how "everything" worked out for the good in Jesus' life. In the light of all this, each of us should try to collaborate with God not only in creation and but also in redemption. We need God's grace and Holy Spirit to overcome our sin, pride and selfishness, and to give us the wisdom and strength to choose and act morally, to love as God calls us (cf. CCC 1999, nn. 385–750; John Paul II 1984 and 1989).

Related to these themes and our topic, Deane-Drummond correctly points out that the reality of human sin, the cross and the future new creation, "where God will be 'all in all,'" counters any naive hope of genetic engineering achieving "utopia on earth" (Deane-Drummond 1995, 319). In discussing the topic of "God's Sovereignty and Genetic Anomalies," Michael Beates says in part that people with genetic anomalies can give glory to God and "show us our own brokenness" and our need of God's grace. "The disabled among us, whether genetically disabled or otherwise, remind us of our own inherent disabilities. When we see them with their limitations, we can begin to see ourselves in a new, more honest manner as broken men and women before God in need of redemption, body and soul" (Beates in Kilner et al. 1997, 53).

In discussing genetics, Rollinson (1999) also speaks of the importance of the incarnation as giving us a benchmark for understanding human nature in a changing world. Jesus, as not only fully divine but also as fully human, is our best model of what it means to be truly human. Jesus gave us an example of loving service, compassion, healing and reaching out to marginalized people. In the Bible there are many instances where God and Jesus show concern for the weak, the sick and the poor (Cole-Turner 1992, 61; cf. CCC 1999, nn. 422–570). Among other things, this is all very relevant to how we treat those suffering from genetic diseases and disabilities.

"Playing God"

The expression "playing God" is often raised in discussions on genetic engineering. What does this mean? The phrase is ambiguous and can be used to mean different things (cf. Hoose 1995, 58). In his enthusiasm for the new genetic technologies,

Joseph Fletcher thinks we should "play God." He thinks we should not fatalistically attribute things to God but take responsibility ourselves. Humanity should use its new powers to control nature, to design and make a better world. Fletcher, however, understands "playing God" in a utilitarian sense, promoting the greatest good for the greatest number of people with little concern for the means used (Fletcher 1974, 200). Many Christians have criticized such an approach, agreeing with the Apostle Paul that we should not do evil to achieve good (cf. Rom 3:8). Paul Ramsey, for example, thinks we should only use genetic technologies in ways that are compatible with human dignity. Among other things, he warns against "playing God" to separate what God has put together, the unitive and procreative goods of human sexuality (consider cloning human beings), or to kill or exploit human beings, even very little ones created in a petri dish, to help others. Ramsey invites us to "play God" in the correct way by imitating God, by honoring and nurturing the nature God gave (Ramsey 1970, 90–96 and 22–52; cf. Verhey in Kilner et al. 1997, 65–68; and Walter 2000, 129–34).

Allen Verhey discusses a few images in the Christian tradition that he thinks are relevant to "playing God" in genetics: God as "creator and healer, and…the one who takes the side of the poor." With regard to God as creator, we are called to appreciate nature and creatively exercise responsible stewardship "in imitation of God's ways, and in service to God's cause." God is also the healer. In his ministry, Jesus often healed people. We, too, are called to promote human life, health and flourishing, and to care for the weak and helpless. With regard to God taking the side of the poor, we are called to try "to mirror God's justice and care for the poor and powerless." Among other things, this includes being concerned for social justice, the fair allocation of resources and the fair distribution of benefits as these relate to the human genome project and genetic powers.

If we are to "play God" as God plays God, then we have a pattern for imitation in God's hospitality to the poor and to the stranger, to the powerless and to the voiceless, to one who is different from both us and the norm, including some genetic norm....[W]e will work for a society where human beings—each of them, even the least of them—is treated as worthy of God's care and affection. (Verhey in Kilner et al. 1997, 69–71. Cf. Matt 25:31–46, which presents Jesus as teaching that what we do to the least human being we do to him; and CCC 1999, nn. 1905–48)

Discussion Questions

1. How do you view plant, animal and human life? Does biological life only have value in terms of its utility for us or does it also have intrinsic value?

2. What are some of the contributions that a Christian perspective can offer to discussions of genetic engineering in a pluralistic society?

3. How do you understand our relationships with nature and God? Should we "play God"?

Chapter Four

Some Concluding Analysis and Reflections

Different ethical conclusions, as well as the choices and actions related to these, can be related to an appreciation or lack of appreciation of certain goods or values. If one's appreciation of the good or valuable is limited to what brings immediate pleasure or enjoyment or what is useful in terms of having one's wants met, then one's ethical conclusions, choices and actions will tend to reflect this. With regard to this we can consider approaches to genetic engineering such as consumerism, maximizing profits, individualism, materialism, maximizing desirable genetic traits and minimizing undesirable genetic defects and their related burdens. Although these approaches can be quite self-centered, they may include some appreciation of values such as autonomy, health, the quality of life and knowledge as these apply to other persons as well. These approaches tend to emphasize freedom of choice with a minimum of ethical standards.

In comparison, some of the ethical conclusions of many Christian ethicists and Catholic teaching might seem to many to be much more restrictive. Genuine Christian ethics, however, can be seen as really very positive and enlightened. It promotes human good or welfare in a complete way. While it appreciates the goods related to the pleasurable and the useful that the above approaches appreciate, it also appreciates what is inherently or intrinsically good. Some goods or values such as the great and equal dignity of every human being regardless of one's capacities, the sacredness of human life, truth, justice, friendship, self-giving love, the marital and procreative meanings of human sexual relations, and fidelity transcend our immediate experience of them and their usefulness for us. Christian teaching that is faithful to the Bible in general and Catholic teaching in particular show a high appreciation for these goods or values.

Respecting such values properly includes not doing certain things that would violate one or more of these values such as aborting unborn human beings including those with disabling diseases, doing non-therapeutic experimentation on human embryos and cloning whole human beings. Choosing such actions would really be counterproductive to human dignity and human good in an integral sense. Choosing actions which fail to respect properly one or more of these values is also counterproductive to our becoming like God (cf. 1 John 3), to our growing in unity and communion with God. This is because ultimately these goods or values are rooted in God who is infinitely good, loving, true, just, faithful and the creator of all life. Since we human beings are created in God's image, failing to respect these goods or values properly also impedes our authentic interpersonal communion with each other. Loving God, oneself and others in a properly ordered way (cf. Matt 22:34–40) includes respecting these goods or values as God does. God loves all that is good in a properly ordered way and we are called to love as he loves (cf. John 15:9–15). God wants to empower us to grow in loving as he loves. This, however, requires each of us to be open to and to cooperate with his grace and Holy Spirit (cf. Rom 5:5; John 14:23–27 and 16:7–15; and Luke 11:9–13). If we do this, we will grow in authentic union and communion with God, each other and the rest of God's creation. Regarding this see, for example, John Paul II (1993); related parts of CCC (1999); and related writings of Christian authors such as Thomas Aquinas and Dietrich von Hildebrand.

If we compare the conclusions of some nonreligious groups with some Christian writers and groups regarding a number of ethical issues related to genetic engineering we will find some areas of widespread agreement. Consider, for example, some of the conclusions presented in Chapter 2 above of the National Bioethics Advisory Commission in the United States (NBAC 1997), Canada's Royal Commission on New Reproductive Technologies (RCNRT 1993), the Church of Scotland (SRT), the Catholic Church (John Paul II, USCC, CHAC, etc.), and a number of Christian writers. One of the reasons for this is that many government and professional groups, and Christian churches and writers, share some common human values related to the physical, psychological and social well-being of people. The classical bioethical principles of beneficence, nonmaleficence, fairness and autonomy are also widely accepted, although not applied in the same ways by everyone. The World, American and Canadian Medical Associations, for example, also include compassion and respect for human dignity/persons in their lists of the principles of medical ethics (see WMA; AMA; and CMA 1996, Preface). There are also some other widely accepted ethical principles or norms related to free and informed consent and confidentiality (cf. Ch. 2.B above; Caulfield 1995), and human research (cf. WMA, "Declaration of Helsinki"; AMA; MRCC et al. 1998; CHAC 2000, VI; Roy et al. 1994, Ch. 13; Ashley and O'Rourke 1997, Chs. 8 and 11.6). Related to these, a few specific areas of widespread (although not universal) agreement with regard to genetic engineering are that: somatic gene therapy and fetal therapy can be ethical for proportionate reasons; and human germ-line gene therapy, human genetic enhancement and human reproductive cloning pose such serious ethical problems that they are either always wrong or at least unethical in the present context.

Examining briefly a few different ethical methods can also be helpful in understanding both areas of disagreement and areas of agreement with regard to specific ethical issues including those related to genetic engineering. Most people and ethicists think it is relevant to consider the consequences of our actions. For example, what are the likely or possible good and bad consequences, both short and long term? Who will benefit and/or suffer? With regard to this, consider many of the hopes and concerns raised above not only regarding the genetic engineering of human beings, but also regarding the genetic engineering of plants and animals (see Chapters 1 and 2 above). Purely consequentialist approaches to ethics reduce ethics to trying to weigh the consequences of actions. If the good consequences outweigh the bad consequences an action is considered moral. Conversely, if the bad consequences outweigh the good consequences an action is considered to be immoral. Consequentialism could be applied selfishly by considering only how one's choices and actions affect oneself and not how they affect others. Some forms of consequentialism, however, are not self-centered—such as utilitarianism which promotes acting for the greatest good for the greatest number of people.

With regard to the morality of human actions, many people also think one's motives or intentions are relevant. For example, is a certain plant or animal being genetically modified with the intention of increasing one's profits and/or to benefit farmers and other people? Is prenatal diagnosis being done with the intention of possible fetal therapy or aborting the fetus if it is found to be 'defective'? Are one's motives self-centered (one only intends to benefit oneself)? Are one's motives related to caring for others (one intends to act in ways that benefit others)? In the teaching of Jesus presented in the Gospels, he criticizes those who did even good things, for example, pray or give alms, with improper motivations, for example, seeking their own praise rather than seeking to please God and respond to the real needs of others (see, e.g., Matt 6:1–6). According to a truly human perspective, we should care not only for our own welfare, but also for the welfare of other human beings. According to an authentic Christian perspective, our motives or intentions should be in accord with loving God, oneself and other human beings, and respecting the rest of God's good creation, in a properly ordered way (cf., e.g., Matt 22:34–40; Gen 1; and Matt 6:26–33).

With regard to the morality of human actions, many people including many Christians also consider whether or not a certain kind of behavior is worthy of our dignity as human beings. Related to some actions is also the question of whether or not they respect the legitimate rights of others. With regard to this consider, for example, some of the discussion in Chapter 2 above with regard to abortion, non-therapeutic experimentation on human embryos, human cloning and sterilization of the mentally handicapped.

Catholic teaching finds common ground with many others in considering the kind of act, one's intention (motives) and the circumstances of an action (which include consequences) to be relevant to the morality of human actions (CCC 1999, nn. 1749–61; John Paul II 1993, nn. 71–83). The most controversial aspect of Catholic moral teaching is that it affirms that some kinds of acts are always wrong to choose, regardless of circumstances or motives. One of the reasons for this conclusion is that choosing some kinds of acts are seen to violate always one or more important personal values/goods such as the intrinsic dignity of human persons, the sacredness of human life, truth and self-giving love. These values are both biblical/Christian values as well as widely appreciated human values. Choosing some kinds of acts cannot be ordered to God, to becoming like God (cf. 1 John 3; Pope John Paul II 1993, n. 78), and to authentic personal communion (see the second and third paragraphs of this chapter above). Some examples relevant to genetic engineering include: the direct killing of innocent human beings including human fetuses and embryos, nontherapeutic experimentation on incompetent human subjects, including living human embryos, dissociating human procreation from loving marital sexual relations (e.g., by in vitro fertilization or cloning human beings) and direct sterilization, whether involuntary or voluntary.

It should be noted here that while Catholic teaching, many ethicists and many other people consider a number of actions to be objectively immoral, this does not mean that we should condemn people who do such actions. With regard to this, we can consider the example of Jesus who disapproved of the sin of the woman caught in adultery but who did not condemn her (John 8:1–11). Among other things, Jesus is reported as saying that he came not to condemn but to save sinners (John 3:17). When a person behaves irresponsibly, his or her subjective culpability can be mitigated, perhaps even eliminated in some cases, by factors that impede his or her free will and/or moral awareness (cf. Luke 12:47–48; and CCC 1999, nn. 1730–1802). Christians believe not only in the truth and justice of God, but also in his mercy. If we have done something that is wrong, we are called to admit this and receive God's healing (cf. 1 John 1:8–9) and to seek reconciliation (cf. much of the New Testament).

It is beyond our purposes here to discuss all ethical methods (see Ashley and O'Rourke 1997, Ch. 7, e.g., for a discussion of some other methods). I would like, however, to add a few comments here with regard to feminist and relational ethics that are relevant to discussions of genetic engineering today. In general, feminists promote the liberation and empowerment of women, which more broadly can be applied to the liberation and empowerment of all human beings. Not all feminists come to the same ethical conclusions with regard to issues related to abortion, genetic engineering and so forth. For example, although many feminists are prochoice with regard to abortion (cf. Wolf 1996), there are also prolife feminists who promote a more consistent life ethics (see, e.g., Chervin 1986). Many feminist and other ethicists speak of the importance of relationships with regard to ethics. It can be easier to make and carry out a good but difficult moral decision if one has some good supportive relationships. For example, it can be easier for a woman to carry a pregnancy to term and to fulfill her responsibilities in raising a child with a genetic disease if she is in a good loving marriage and has a good supportive social network. One of the insights of a good "relational ethics" is that it is important not only to discern correctly regarding the morality of human actions; it is also important to support people to choose and act morally by assisting them in appropriate ways according to their needs.

As we move into the biotech century, Jeremy Rifkin says we face a dilemma and difficult choices: part of us "reels at the prospect of further desacralizing of life, of reducing ourselves and all other sentient creatures to chemical codes to be manipulated for purely instrumental and utilitarian ends"; another side of us is committed to progress—"Not to proceed with this revolution is unthinkable..." (Rifkin 1998, 169–70; cf. James Watson in *Time* 1999, 71). Technology extends human power that is not neutral. Will genetic engineering result in more good than harm? Will it lead to more or less respect for life? The question is not whether or not to use technology, but which ones. Society may choose to use some biotechnologies (e.g., genetic screening of diseases that can be treated early and gene-splicing for life-saving pharmaceutical products) and not others (e.g., human germ-line therapy and genetic enhancement, and releasing large numbers of transgenic organisms into the biosphere). Rifkin favors a conservative ecological approach that may include using some genetic engineering such as somatic gene therapy to ward off seriously debilitating or deadly diseases where holistic and preventative health are insufficient. He and others such as Dr. Donald Bruce call for a wide debate and conversation, with each of us taking responsibility, that is, not just scientists and corporate managers but also consumers and ordinary people (Rifkin 1998, 231–34; and SRT).

Such a conversation, I think, will be more fruitful if it is linked to an appropriate education. With regard to this, consider the following statement by Pope John Paul II. He speaks of the urgent need for an education in ecological responsibility:

> This education cannot be rooted in mere sentiment or empty wishes. Its purpose cannot be ideological or political. It must

not be based on a rejection of the modern world or a vague desire to return to some "paradise lost." Instead, a true education in responsibility entails a genuine conversion in ways of thought and behavior. Churches and religious bodies, non-governmental and governmental organizations, indeed all members of society, have a precise role to play in such education. The first educator, however, is the family, where the child learns to respect his neighbor and to love nature. (John Paul II 1989, n. 13)

Schools and other institutions of education, the various media and self-education can also play important roles in such an education.

Discussion Questions

1. What are some areas of widespread agreement today with regard to genetic engineering? What issues are quite controversial? With regard to these issues, what values do you consider important, most important? Are there any values that you think we should respect in all situations?

2. Do you agree with the Catholic approach to morality that we should consider not only consequences and motives, but also the kind of act and whether or not it can be ordered to God and a proper respect for human dignity? In what ways are other ethical approaches or methods similar or different?

3. How can each of us contribute to developing good relationships and fostering the kind of education that will promote good moral living including being ecologically responsible?

References

[AMA] American Medical Association web site: <http://www.americanmedicalassociation.org/>.

Asch, Adrienne, and Gail Geller. 1996. "Feminism, bioethics, and genetics." *Feminism & bioethics: beyond reproduction,* 318–50, ed. Susan M. Wolf. New York: Oxford University Press.

Ashley, Benedict. 1985. *Theologies of the body: Humanist and Christian.* Braintree, Mass.: The Pope John XXIII Medical-Moral Research and Education Center.

Ashley, Benedict, and Kevin O'Rourke. 1994. *Ethics of health care: An introductory textbook.* 2nd ed. Washington, D.C.: Georgetown University Press.

Ashley, Benedict, and Kevin O'Rourke. 1997. *Health care ethics: A theological analysis.* 4th ed. Washington, D.C.: Georgetown University Press.

Barnard, Jeff. 1999, Sept. 2. "Baby Einsteins next? Talk about building a better mousetrap; this gene experiment created smarter mice." *Edmonton Journal* A1.

[Bill C-47] House of Commons of Canada. 1996, June 14. "Bill C-47: First reading." Ottawa: Canada Communication Group Publishing. This bill never became law.

BioNews. "Search the BioNews Archive": <http://www.progress.org.uk/News/BioNewsSearch.html>.

Branswell, Helen. 1998, Dec. 9. "Cloning plan raises spectre of farms for human organs." *Edmonton Journal* A8.

Breckenridge, Joan. 1987, Sept. 23. "Clinic improves chances of choosing child's sex." *Globe and Mail* A1–2.

Bruce, Donald, and Ann Bruce, eds. 1998. *Engineering genesis: The ethics of genetic engineering in non-human species.* London: Earthscan Publications Limited.

Bryannan, Laura. 1999, Feb. "Dangers of genetic screening." <http://homestar.org/bryannan/genetic.html>.

Bueckert, Dennis. 1999, Apr. 30. "Canada leads move to set standards on genetic foods." *Edmonton Journal* A12.

Burnett, Sterling. 2000, May 16. "Genetically modified foods vital to feed a growing population." *Edmonton Journal* A15.

Cairney, Richard. 1998, Sept. 18. "Renegade researchers intent on xenotransplants." *Folio* (University of Alberta), 6.

Callahan, Daniel. 1997, Sept.–Oct. "Cloning: The work not done." *Hastings Center Report* 18–20.

Canadian Conference of Catholic Bishops Executive. 1996, Oct. 15. "Position of the Canadian Conference of Catholic Bishops on Bill C-47: The Human Reproductive and Genetic Technologies Act." <http//www.cam.org/~cccb/html_declaration_publiques/1996_nov-b_e.htm>.

Canadian Institute of Health Research. 2001. *Human stem cell research: Opportunities for health and ethical perspectives: A discussion paper.* Ottawa: Public Works and Government Services.

Catholic News Service. 1998, Jan. 19. "Theologians reject cloning plans." *Western Catholic Reporter* 5.

Caulfield, Timothy. 1995. "The practice of human genetics: emerging areas of consensus?" *Health Law Journal* 3:307–20.

CBC [Canadian Broadcasting Corporation]. 1992. *On the eighth day, part 2: Perfecting mother nature* (video). Directed by

Gwynne Basen. Coproduced by Mary Armstrong, CBC, National Film Board and Cinefort Inc., Montreal.

[CCC] John Paul II. 1999. *Catechism of the Catholic Church*. Revised Edition. Ottawa: Canadian Conference of Catholic Bishops.

[CDF] Congregation for the Doctrine of the Faith. 1987. *Instruction on respect for human life in its origin and on the dignity of procreation [Donum Vitae]*. Boston: Daughters of St. Paul.

[CHAC] Catholic Health Association of Canada. 1991. *Health care ethics guide*. Ottawa: Author.

[CHAC] Catholic Health Association of Canada. 2000. *Health ethics guide*. Ottawa: Author.

Chambers, Allan. 2001, Feb. 2. "Cut through 'geno-hype' over cloning, law professor says." *Edmonton Journal* A3.

[CHAUSA] Catholic Health Association of the United States. 1990. *Human genetics: Ethical issues in genetic testing, counseling and therapy*. St. Louis, Mo.: Author. The CHAUSA web site <http://www.chausa.org/> also has many articles online from Health Progress and other sources related to genetics and ethical issues. See their "Search" tool.

Chervin, Ronda. 1986. *Feminine, free and faithful*. San Francisco: Ignatius Press.

Childress, James. 1997, Sept.–Oct. "The Challenges of Public Ethics." *Hastings Center Report* 9–11.

[CMA] Canadian Medical Association. 1996. *Code of Ethics of the Canadian Medical Association*. <http://www.cma.ca/inside/policybase/1996/10-15.htm>.

Cole-Turner, R. 1992. "Religion and the Human Genome." *Journal of Religion and Health* 31:2.

Colleton, Michael. 1993, March. "The Human Genome Project: Some ethical considerations." In *Trends in Bioethics,* Edmonton: St. Joseph's College Catholic Bioethics Centre.

Cornwell, John. 1995, May 27. "Ourselves and our genes." *The Tablet* 656–58.

Deane-Drummond, Celia E. 1995, July. "Genetic engineering for the environment: Ethical implications of the biotechnology revolution." *The Heythrop Journal* 36:307–27.

DeMarco, Donald. 1987. *In my mother's womb: The Catholic Church's defense of natural life.* Manassas, Va.: Trinity Communications.

DiCenzo, David. 2000, Mar. 17. "Modifying the genetically modified foods debate." *Folio* (University of Alberta) 3.

Dixon, Patrick. 1993. *The genetic revolution.* Eastbourne: Kingsway.

Doerflinger, Richard M. 1999. "The ethics of funding embryonic stem cell research: A Catholic viewpoint." *Kennedy Institute of Ethics Journal* 9:137–50.

[EB] *The New Encyclopedia Britannica: Macropaedia.* 1975. 30 vols. London: Encyclopedia Britannica, Inc.

Edmonton Journal Editorial. 1998, Jan. 14. "Hello Dolly, Goodbye Dr. Seed." *Edmonton Journal* A8.

Elliott, Lee. 1998, Sept. 18. "Can genetic researchers be trusted with the gene pool?: Examining the implications for people with disabilities." *Folio* (University of Alberta) 6.

Elliott, Lee, and Richard Cairney. 1998, Sept. 18. "Whose drum are you marching to? …new pressures researchers face as commerce enters the lab." *Folio* (University of Alberta) 3.

[ELSI] The National Human Genome Research Institute's Ethical, Legal, and Social Implications Program web site: <http://www.nhgri.nih.gov/ELSI/>.

Engelhardt, H. Tristram, Jr. 1999, Aug. "Genetic enhancement and theosis: Two models of therapy." *Christian Bioethics* 197–99.

[FDA] The United States Food and Drug Administration web site: <http://www.fda.gov/>.

Filteau, Jerry. 2001, Aug. 20. "Bush stem-cell plan promotes complicity in evil—theologian." *Western Catholic Reporter* 5.

Flaman, Paul. 2001, Summer. "The ethics of cloning plants, animals, human beings and embryos." *Journal: A Publication of the Canadian Chapter Fellowship of Catholic Scholars Amicale Des Savants Catholiques* 3–11. This article was adapted from an earlier draft of sections 1.D and 2.E of this book.

Fletcher, Joseph. 1974. *The ethics of genetic control: Ending reproductive roulette.* Garden City, N.Y.: Anchor Books.

Frazier O'Brien, Nancy. 2001, Aug. 20. "U.S. Bishops deplore Bush's stem cell stand." *Western Catholic Reporter* 1.

Gattaca. 1997. Movie directed by John R. Woodward. Columbia Pictures.

GeneClinics online: <http://www.geneclinics.org/>. See also their companion site GeneTests online: http://www.genetests.org/>.

Geron Ethics Advisory Board. 1999, Mar.–Apr. "Research with human embryonic stem cells: ethical considerations." *Hastings Center Report* 31–36.

Golden, Frederic. 1999, Jan. 11. "Good eggs, bad eggs." *Time* 40–43.

Gonzalez, Ramon. 1997, Mar. 3. "Quit cloning around: Cloned sheep raises spectre of manufactured humans." *Western Catholic Reporter* 1 and 3.

Gustafson, James. 1984. *Ethics from a theocentric perspective.* Chicago: University of Chicago Press.

Harris, John. 1992. *Wonderwoman and superman: The ethics of human biotechnology.* New York: Oxford University Press.

Health Canada. 2001, May. *Proposals for legislation governing assisted human reproduction: An overview.* Ottawa: Health Canada.

Hellen, Nicholas. 2000, Mar. 5. "Scientists hope to clone 'zoo' of extinct animals." *Edmonton Journal* A3.

[HGP Information] Human Genome Project Information. 2000. <http://www.ornl.gov/hgmis/about.html>.

Hoose, Bernard. 1995, January. "Ethics and genetics." *The Way* 35:55–62.

Hubbard, Ruth, and Elijah Wald. 1993. *Exploding the gene myth.* Boston: Beacon Press.

Humber, James, and Robert Almeder. 1998. *Human cloning.* Atlanta: Georgia State University.

Indigenous Peoples. 1995, Feb. 19. "Declaration of Indigenous Peoples of the Western Hemisphere regarding the Human Genome Diversity Project." Phoenix, Arizona. <http://www.anatomy.su.oz.au/danny/anthropology/anthro-I/archive/february-1995/0809.html>.

Jick, Bryan, M.D. 1999, May. "Gender selection: The latest techniques for choosing the sex of your child." <http://www.parenthoodweb.com/parent_cfmfiles/pros.cfm/839>.

John Paul II. 1981. Apostolic exhortation *Familiaris consortio* "The role of the Christian family in the modern world." Boston: St. Paul Editions.

John Paul II. 1983, Dec. 5. "Dangers of genetic manipulation: Address to members of the World Medical Association, October 29, 1983." *L'Osservatore Romano* 10–11.

John Paul II. 1984. *On the Christian meaning of human suffering.* Boston: Pauline Books and Media.

John Paul II. 1989, Dec. 8. *The ecological crisis: A common responsibility.* Washington, D.C.: United States Catholic Conference.

John Paul II. 1993. Encyclical letter *Veritatis splendor* regarding certain fundamental questions of the church's moral teaching. Ottawa: Canadian Conference of Catholic Bishops.

John Paul II. 1995a. "The human person—beginning and end of scientific research" (Address to the Pontifical Academy of Science, 28 October 1994), *The Pope Speaks* (March–April) 40:80–84.

John Paul II. 1995b. Encyclical letter *Evangelium vitae* "The Gospel of life." Sherbrooke, QC: Médiaspaul.

John Paul II. 1998. Encyclical letter *Fides et ratio* on the relationship between faith and reason. Ottawa: Canadian Conference of Catholic Bishops.

John Paul II. 2000, Aug. 30. "Holy Father to Transplant Congress." *L'Osservatore Romano* (English edition) 2.

Junker-Kenny, Maureen, and Lisa Sowle Cahill. 1998. *The ethics of genetic engineering.* London: SCM Press.

Kaveny, M. Cathleen. 1999, March. "Jurisprudence and genetics." *Theological Studies* 135–47.

Keenan, James, S.J. 1999, Aug. "Whose perfection is it anyway?: A virtuous consideration of enhancement." *Christian Bioethics* 104–20.

Kilner, John F., Rebecca D. Pentz, and Frank E. Young, eds. 1997. *Genetic ethics: Do the ends justify the genes?* Grand Rapids: William B Eerdmans.

Klotzko, Arlene Judith, J.D. 1997. "A report from America: The debate about Dolly." *Bioethics* 11:5:427–38.

Kmiec, Eric. 1999, May–June. "Gene therapy." *American Scientist.* <http://www.amsci.org/amsci/articles/99articles/Kmiec.html>.

Knox, Richard. 1999, Feb. 1. "AIDS virus traced to chimps." *Edmonton Journal* A1 and A14.

Kotulak, Ronald. 1997, Feb. 24. "Scientists clone lamb. Will humans be next?" *Edmonton Journal* A1 and A16.

Lanza, Robert P., Jose B. Cibelli, Catherine Blackwell, Vincent J. Cristofalo, Mary Kay Francis, Gabriela M. Baerlocher, Jennifer Mak, Michael Schertzer, Elizabeth A. Chavez, Nancy Sawyer, Peter M. Lansdorp, and Michael D. West. 2000, Apr. 28. "Extension of Cell Life-Span and Telomere Length in Animals Cloned from Senescent Somatic Cells." *Science* 665-69.

Lejeune, Jerome. 1991. "Genes and human life: Testimony given to the Louisiana State Legislature on June 7, 1990." <http://www.ewtn.com/library/PROLIFFE/GENESLIF.TXT>.

Lemonick, Michael D. 1998, Nov. 16. "The biological mother lode." *Time* 74–75.

Linn, Matthew and Dennis, S.J., and Sheila Fabricant. 1985. *At Peace with the unborn: A book of healing.* New York: Paulist Press.

[LRCC] Law Reform Commission of Canada. 1979. *Sterilization: Implications for mentally retarded and mentally ill persons.* Ottawa: Author.

May, William E. 1977. *Human existence, medicine and ethics.* Chicago: Franciscan Herald Press.

May, William E. 2000. *Catholic Bioethics and the gift of human life.* Huntington: Our Sunday Visitor.

McGee, Glenn. 1997. "Ethical issues in genetics in the next 100 years: Lecture presented to the UNESCO Asian Bioethics Congress." (November 6). <http://www.med.upenn.edu/~bioethic/ genetics/articles/3.mcgee.kobe.html>.

Moltmann, Jürgen. 1985. *God in creation: An ecological doctrine of creation.* Translated by Margaret Kohl. SCM Press Ltd.

[MRCC] Medical Research Council of Canada. 1990. "Guidelines for research on somatic cell gene therapy in humans." In *Readings in biomedical ethics: A Canadian focus,* ed. E. H. Kluge. Scarborough: Prentice Hall (1993) 515–22.

[MRCC et al.] Medical Research Council of Canada, Natural Sciences and Engineering Research Council of Canada, and Social Sciences and Humanities Research Council of Canada. 1998. *Tri-council policy statement: Ethical conduct for research involving humans.* Ottawa: Medical Research Council of Canada.

Munson, R., and L.H. Davis. 1992. "Germ-line gene therapy and the medical imperative." *Kennedy Institute of Ethics Journal* 2:137–58.

Murphy, Timothy F., and Marc A. Lappé, ed. 1994. *Justice and the Human Genome Project*. Berkeley: University of California Press.

Nash, J. Madeleine. 1998, Feb. 9. "The case for cloning." *Time* 50.

NativeNet. 1998. "Human Genome Diversity Project articles from NATIVE-L." <http://bioc09.uthscsa.edu.natnet/archive/nlhddp.html>.

[NBAC] National Bioethics Advisory Commission. 1997, June. "Executive summary from *Cloning human beings: The report and recommendations of the National Bioethics Advisory Commission.*" *Hastings Center Report* (Sept.–Oct. 1997) 7–9.

[NBAC] National Bioethics Advisory Commission web site: <http://www.bioethics.gov>.

[NFB] National Film Board of Canada. 1986. "Who should decide? Prenatal diagnosis." *Discussions in bioethics* (video). Montreal: Author.

[NFB] National Film Board of Canada. 1996. *The sterilization of Leilani Muir* (video). Montreal: Author.

[NIH] United States National Institutes of Health web site: <http://www.nih.gov>.

[NSGC] National Society of Genetic Counselors, Inc. 1992. *Code of Ethics.* <http://www.nsgc.org/ethicsCode.html>.

O'Callaghan, John. 1994. "Genetic engineering: Ethical considerations." *Topics in bioethics for science and religion teachers.* Edmonton Catholic Schools and St. Albert Catholic Schools.

Option X beginning now: Explorations into genetics and bioethics. 1998. A Senior High Science Resource; Interactive CD-ROM with teacher's guide. Edmonton: The Redemptorist Bioethics Consultancy of Canada.

Paul VI. 1968. Encyclical letter *Humanae vitae* "Of human life." Boston: St. Paul Editions.

Pius XI. 1930. Encyclical letter on Christian marriage *Casti connubii*. Boston: St. Paul Editions.

Polkinghorne, John. 1998. *Science and theology*. Minneapolis: Fortress Press.

[RAFI] Rural Advancement Foundation International. 1999, Mar. 29. "Traitor technology: 'Damaged goods' from the gene giants." <http://www.rafi.org/pr/release30.html>.

Ramsey, Paul. 1970. *Fabricated man: The ethics of genetic control*. New Haven and London: Yale University Press.

[RCNRT] Royal Commission on New Reproductive Technologies. 1993. *Proceed with care: The final report of the Royal Commission on New Reproductive Technologies*. Ottawa: Canada Communications Group Publishing. In this book references are to the "Summary of main topics."

Reuters. 1999, Oct. 21. "Breakthrough in artificial chromosomes." *Edmonton Journal* A3.

Reuters. 2000, Feb. 29. "Multinational control of biotechnology condemned." *Edmonton Journal* A14.

Reuters. 2000, Apr. 28. "Cloned cows 'reset' aging clock." *Edmonton Journal* A5.

Rifkin, Jeremy. 1998. *The biotech century: Harnessing the gene and remaking the world*. New York: Jeremy P. Torcher/Putran.

Riga, Peter J. 1998, August. "Doctors, culture and genetic counselling." *Linacre Quarterly* 48–51.

Ritter, Malcolm. 2001, Feb. 11. "Studies find fewer human genes than thought." *Edmonton Journal* A5.

Rodriguez, Eduardo. 1998, May. "The Human Genome Project and eugenics." *Linacre Quarterly* 73–81.

Rodriguez, Eduardo. 2000, Feb. "Social attitudes and the Human Genome Project: Ethical implications." *Linacre Quarterly* 28–40.

Rogers, Lois. 2000, May 14. "Cloned animals developing tumors and other diseases." *Edmonton Journal* A3.

Rollinson, Andrew. 1999, Mar. *A Christian perspective on genetics.* <http://www.christian.org.uk/genetics.htm>.

Rosner, Fred, M.D. 1991. *Modern medicine and Jewish ethics.* New York: Yeshiva University Press.

Roy, David J., John R. Williams, and Bernard M. Dickens. 1994. *Bioethics in Canada.* Scarborough, Ontario: Prentice Hall Canada Inc.

Science Council of Canada. 1991. *Genetics in Canadian health care.* Ottawa: Author.

Shannon, Thomas A. 2000, Mar. "Ethical issues in genetics." *Theological Studies* 111–23.

[SRT] Church of Scotland. *Society, Religion and Technology Project.* <http://dspace.dial.pipex.com/srtscot/srtpage3.shtml>. SRT's site has about 100 Web pages on genetic engineering and other topics. Specific references in the text will include the date accessed and the name of the article.

Stephenson, J. 1995, June 21. "Terms of engraftment: Umbilical cord blood transplants arouse enthusiasm." *JAMA: The Journal of the American Medical Association* 1813–15.

Sterling, Burnett. 2000, May 16. "Genetically Modified Foods Vital to Feed a Growing Population." *Edmonton Journal* A 15.

Supreme Court of Canada. 1986, Oct. "Eve v. Mrs. E." *Readings in biomedical ethics: A Canadian focus,* ed. Eike-Henner Kluge. Scarborough: Prentice Hall Canada Inc. (1993) 412–18.

Sutton, Agneta. 1995, August. "The new genetics: Facts, fictions and fears." *Linacre Quarterly* 76–87.

Suzuki, David, and Peter Knudtson. 1988. *Genethics: The ethics of engineering life.* Toronto: Stoddart Publishing Co. Limited.

Thavis, John. 1999, Oct. 18. "Vatican experts OK some biotechnology but they say no to human cloning." *Western Catholic Reporter* (Edmonton), 1 and 5. See also "On File." *Origins* (Oct. 21, 1999) 294.

The Associated Press. 1997, Oct. 19. "Headless frog embryo moves human cloning step closer." *Edmonton Journal* A11.

The Associated Press. 1999, Sept. 30. "Gene therapy test halted after man, 18, with rare disease dies." *Edmonton Journal* A5.

The Associated Press. 2000, Nov. 7. "Cadavers yield valuable stem cells." *Edmonton Journal* A15.

The Associated Press London. 2001, Jan. 23. "Lords back embryo cloning." *Edmonton Journal* A9.

The Canadian Press. 1999, Aug. 31. "'Molecular farming' wave of future." *Edmonton Journal* A3.

Time (Canadian Edition). 1999, Jan. 11. "Special issue: The future of medicine: How genetic engineering will change us in the next century." 26–71.

Thorne, Duncan. 2001, Feb. 1. "Nothing wrong with human cloning, says U of A ethicist." *Edmonton Journal* A1.

[UNESCO] United Nations Educational, Scientific and Cultural Organization. 1997, Nov. 11. "Universal declaration on the human genome and human rights." Available online: <http://www.unesco.org/opi/29gencon/egenkit.htm>.

Unland, Karen. 1999, Apr. 11. "Ethics critical in finding genetic basis of illness." *Edmonton Journal* A10.

Urdang, Laurence, and Helen Harding Swallow, eds. 1983. *Mosby's Medical and Nursing Dictionary.* Toronto: The C. V. Mosby Company.

[USCC] United States Conference of Catholic Bishops. 1994. "Ethical and religious directives for Catholic health care services." *Origins: CNS Documentary Service* (15 Dec. 1994) 449–62.

[USCC] United States Conference of Catholic Bishops. 1996. *Critical decisions: Genetic testing and its implications.* Washington, D.C.: United States Catholic Conference. Available online: <http://www.nccbuscc.org/shv/testing.htm>.

[USCC] United States Conference of Catholic Bishops. 2000, Jan. 31. "Bishops' conference comments on NIH guidelines for embryonic stem cell research." Letter to NIH Office of Science Policy by Rev. Msgr. Dennis N. Schnurr, General Secretary on behalf of the USCC. Available online: <http://www.nccbuscc.org/prolife/issues/bioethic/comments.htm>.

Vanier, Jean. 1985. *Man and woman he made them.* New York: Paulist Press.

Varga, Andrew. 1984. *The main issues in bioethics.* Revised edition. New York: Paulist Press.

Walter, James J. 2000, Mar. "Theological issues in genetics." *Theological Studies* 124–34.

Weiss, Rick. 1998, Dec. 9. "Cattle cloners making themselves herd." *Edmonton Journal* A1.

Weiss, Rick. 2000, Oct. 15. "Birth of human cloning?" *Edmonton Journal* A3.

Wevrick, Rachel. 1999, Jul. 6. "Genetic engineering": e-mail from <rachel.wevrick@ualberta.ca to pflaman@ualberta.ca>. Dr. Wevrick is a professor with the Department of Medical Genetics, at the University of Alberta, in Edmonton, Canada.

Wilkie, Tom. 1998, Aug. 1. "We reap what we sow: ...genetically manipulating food...." *The Tablet* 995–96.

Williams, John R. 1997. "The churches and genetics." *Christian perspectives on bioethics,* Ch. 5. Ottawa: Novalis.

Wilmut, Ian. 1999, Jan. 11. "Dolly's false legacy." *Time* (Canadian Edition) 52–55.

Wilson, James. 1999, May. "Human gene therapy." The Institute for Human Gene Therapy, University of Pennsylvania. <http://www.med.upenn.edu/ihgt/info/prospcts.html>.

Wooden, Cindy. 2001, July 16. "Scientist, Vatican agree on genetically modified foods." Catholic News Service Rome as reprinted in *Western Catholic Reporter* 5.

[WMA] World Medical Association web site: <http://www.wma.net>.

Wolf, Susan M., ed. 1996. *Feminism & bioethics: Beyond reproduction.* New York: Oxford University Press.

Yoon, Carol Kaesuk. 2000, May 1. "These pharm animals boggle the mind." *Edmonton Journal* A3.

Zenit News Agency. 2001, Sept. 26. "Animal-to-man organ transplants deemed OK under right conditions: Vatican outlines position in special document." <http://www.zenit.org>.

Suggested Reading / Viewing

Catholic Health Association of the United States web site: <http://www.chausa.org>. This site has many articles from *Health Progress* and other sources online related to genetics and ethical issues. See their "Search" tool.

[CBC] Canadian Broadcasting Corporation. 1992. *On the eighth day, Part 2: Perfecting mother nature* (video). Directed by Gwynne Basen. Coproduced by Mary Armstrong, CBC, National Film Board and Cinefort Inc., Montreal.

Church of Scotland. 1998. *Society, Religion and Technology Project* [SRT]. <http://dspace.dial.pipex.com/srtscot/srtpage3. shtml>. SRT's site has more than 100 Web pages on genetic engineering and other topics.

Congregation for the Doctrine of the Faith. 1987. *Instruction on respect for human life in its origin and on the dignity of procreation [Donum vitae]*. Boston: Daughters of St. Paul.

Gattaca. 1997. Movie directed by John R. Woodward. Columbia Pictures.

John Paul II. 1983, Dec. 5. "Dangers of genetic manipulation: Address to members of the World Medical Association, October 29, 1983." *L'Osservatore Romano* 10–11.

John Paul II. 1995. Encyclical letter *Evangelium vitae* "The Gospel of life." Sherbrooke, QC: Médiaspaul.

Kilner, John F., Rebecca D. Pentz, and Frank E. Young, eds. 1997. *Genetic Ethics: Do the Ends Justify the Genes?* Grand Rapids: William B Eerdmans.

[NFB] National Film Board of Canada. 1986. "Who should decide? Prenatal diagnosis." *Discussions in bioethics* (video). Montreal: Author.

Option X beginning now: Explorations into genetics and bioethics. 1998. A Senior High Science Resource; Interactive CD-ROM with teacher's guide. Edmonton: The Redemptorist Bioethics Consultancy of Canada.

Rifkin, Jeremy. 1998. *The biotech century: Harnessing the gene and remaking the world.* New York: Jeremy P. Torcher/Putran.

Index